ELECTROCARDIOGRAPHIC ATLAS

HENNING GØTZSCHE

ELECTROCARDIOGRAPHIC

ATLAS

First English Edition

AN F.A.D.L.s FORLAG PUBLICATION
Distributed by
Year Book Medical Publishers, Inc.
35 E. Wacker Drive, Chicago

Original Danish Editions
© 1967 and 1973 by F.A.D.L.s Forlag
English Edition
© 1976 by F.A.D.L.s Forlag
Translated from the Danish by Harry Cowan, B.Sc.
This book is copyrighted in Denmark and may not be
reproduced by any means in whole or in part without written
permission from the copyright owner.
Distributed throughout the world except for Denmark, Norway,
Finland and Sweden by Year Book Medical Publishers, Inc.
Library of Congress Catalog Card Number: 74-29350
ISBN: 0 8151-3825-3
Printed in Denmark
by Th. Laursens Bogtrykkeri a-s, Tønder

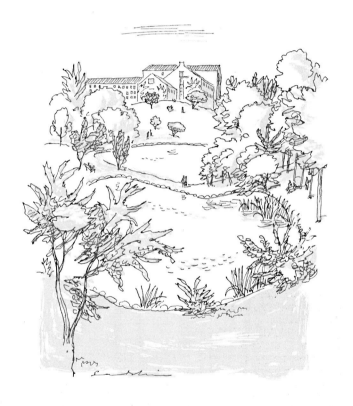

University of Århus
Denmark

CONTENTS

PREFACE

The aim of this book is to make available to students and young doctors a pocket book-size collection of characteristic electrocardiograms, illustrating all common and a few less common patterns.

The main section of the book (pp. 31–149) is an atlas. This is so arranged that each double page describes only one subject or a part of one subject. Each double page has pictures on the left page and the corresponding descriptive text on the right with easily recognizable numbering. Introducing each subject is a short survey of concepts and definitions.

The first part of the book contains a simple guide to evaluating electrocardiograms for the beginner (pp. 11–22) and a glossary of terms in common use in the description of cardiac dysrhythmias (pp. 23-30)

Finally, a collection of exercises in evaluating electrocardiograms is included in the last part of the book.

The text is purely descriptive. Physiologic and pathologic aspects and correlations should be sought in current textbooks.

Some of the illustrations are marked with an asterisk (*) after the figure number, denoting that the example is considered less important to health service personnel on a more basic training level. Such marking is a rough estimate, and will thus be open to criticism, but I hope that it will help inexperienced students and nurses in using the atlas.

It should be noted that the standard time marking – if not otherwise indicated on the curves – is 50 mm/second, cf. page 13.

Henning Gøtzsche

PRACTICAL GUIDANCE IN EVALUATING ELECTROCARDIOGRAMS

For the untrained student, some schematic procedure can be helpful in interpreting electrocardiograms. For example, the following scheme might be chosen.

(1) Rhythm.
(2) Rate.
(3) P waves.
(4) P-R interval.
(5) The QRS complex:
  (a) Duration.
  (b) Configuration.
  (c) Electrical axis.
(6) S-T segment.
(7) T waves.
(8) U waves.
(9) Q-T interval.

The individual points will be discussed in the following.

(1) Rhythm.

By *regular rhythm* usually is understood regular ventricular rhythm.

Regular rhythm thus implies
equal R-R intervals.

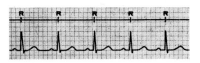

Note whether it is a case of

normal sinus rhythm

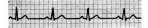

or of a regular ectopic rhythm, either from the atria

in atrial paroxysmal tachycardia

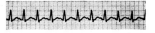

and some cases of atrial flutter

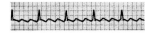

or from the atrioventricular junction
(junctional rhythm)

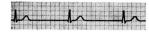

or from a center in the
ventricles
(idioventricular rhythm).

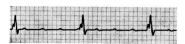

In *arrhythmia,* it should be noted whether there is *a certain degree of system* in the irregularity, e.g., the normal

respiratory sinus arrhythmia

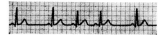

or
coupled extrasystoles
(here, junctional)

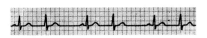

or Wenckebach periods

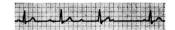

or whether the arrhythmia appears *quite random,* e.g., in

sinoatrial block,

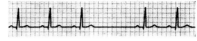

or in scattered extrasystoles

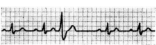

or whether there is *complete irregularity*

as in atrial fibrillation.

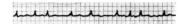

(2) Rate.

In clinical electrocardiography two standardized paper speeds are in general use: 50 mm/second, common in Scandinavia, and 25 mm/second, common in Anglo-Saxon countries,

so that the interval between two heavily drawn vertical lines is 0.1 second (at 50 mm/second) resp. 0.2 second (at 25 mm/second), and between two fine vertical lines 0.2 second (at 50 mm/second) resp. 0.04 second (at 25 mm/second).

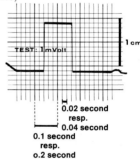

The ventricular rate then is determined by counting the number of "large" intervals between two R waves and dividing this into 600 (as 600×0.1 second = 1 minute) in " Scandinavian" tracings:

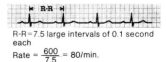

resp. into 300 (as 300×0.2 second = 1 minute) in tracings with the slower paper speed.

13

The atrial rate is determined in a similar manner by counting the number of "large" intervals between two P waves and dividing this into 600 resp. 300.

In case of arrhythmia, a mean value is of course taken.

NB: In this atlas, a time marking is inserted on the tracings only in cases where the ordinary "Scandinavian" (50 mm/second) is not used.

(3) P waves.

The tracing should be inspected to determine whether there is a P wave for each QRS complex, and the shape, duration and amplitude of the P wave is noted.

In hypertrophy and dilatation of the right atrium, the P waves become tall and narrow.

In left atrial enlargement, the P waves become wide and often notched.

Too many P waves in relation to the number of QRS complexes are seen, for example, in

atrioventicular block

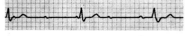

and in atrial flutter ("F waves")

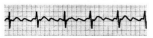

and often in atrial fibrillation ("f waves").

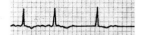

Too few P waves in relation to the number of QRS complexes often are seen in atrioventricular dissociation; e.g.,

atrioventricular
dissociation with
interference.

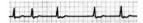

Absence of P waves in more leads can be seen in

atrial fibrillation.

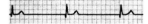

In atrial fibrillation, however, there will as a rule – at any rate periodically –

be visible P waves ("f waves") in the
right precordial leads
(V_1 and V_2).

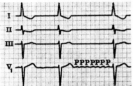

Absence of P waves often is due to the P waves being hidden within the QRS complexes; e.g.,

in some cases of junctional rhythm.

Ectopic P waves deviate in shape from those arising from the sinoatrial node, and often are designated P'.

(4) P-R interval.

P-R interval = P-Q interval is measured from the beginning of the P wave to the beginning of the QRS complex. The measurement is made in the lead (including the precordial leads) in which the interval is greatest.

The P-R interval normally is not above 0.22 second (some say 0.20 second). The P-R interval normally is shorter in children, and it also varies with rate.

Prolonged P-R interval is seen in

first degree atrioventricular block.

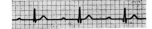

Shortened P-R interval (i.e., less than 0.12 second) is seen in

simple pre-excitation

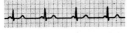

and in the W-P-W syndrome

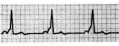

and in some cases of junctional rhythm (here, retrograde conduction).

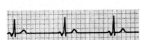

(5) QRS complex.

The waves in this complex are defined as follows:

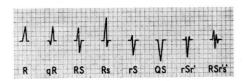

The Q wave is the first deflection in the complex if it is negative. The R wave is the first positive wave. The S wave is a negative deflection following the R wave. If the QRS complex consists of only one negative deflection, this negative wave is called a QS wave. If there are two or more positive waves, these are designated R, R′, R″, etc., and the negative waves after these are designated S, S′, S″, etc. Capital and small letters often are used to indicate the pattern.

16

The *duration* of the QRS complex is measured in that lead in which it is greatest. The QRS duration usually is regarded as normal when it is less than 0.10 second. Increased duration of QRS is seen

in bundle branch block

0.15 second

and in idioventricular rhythm.

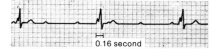
0.16 second

With regard to the *configuration* of the QRS complex, it should first be noted whether it is constant or varying. Small periodic changes are observed in changes in the position of the heart

during respiration.

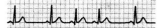

Slight irregularities in the shape are seen as a result of superimposition of atrial waves in atrial flutter

and atrial fibrillation.

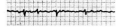

A somewhat varying shape is also seen in some ectopic ventricular rhythms, especially

ventricular tachycardia.

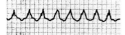

A quite deviant shape of one or more QRS complexes suggests discharge from various foci, and is most commonly seen in

ventricular extrasystoles

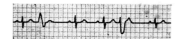

and in escape beats, and is also seen in

atrial arrest with
multifocal idioventri-
cular rhythm.

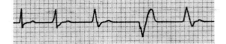

Even more bizarre QRS complexes are seen in

ventricular
fibrillation.

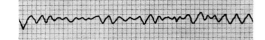

An evaluation of *the electrical axis,* i.e., the mean axis of the QRS complex, is of significance, especially in sinus rhythm. This evaluation often provides some over-all description of the configuration in the standard leads I, II and III. Axis evaluation is illustrated on pages 41-43.

The most important normal values for QRS are shown in the tables on page 33. Pathologic QRS complexes are of great significance for evaluating myocardial disease. The most important pathologic patterns are described in what follows.

(6) S-T segment.

Note is taken whether the S-T segment, i.e., the segment from the end of the QRS complex to the start of the T wave, deviates from the isoelectric line. By definition, the isoelectric line is the level of the segment from the T wave (or the U wave) to the P wave in the following beat,

i.e., the T-P interval:

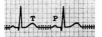

In some cases, e.g., in tachycardia, this interval is not well defined, and we then use

18

the level immediately before the QRS
complex as the isoelectric line.

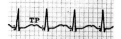

Normally, the S-T segment does not deviate more than 1 mm (= 0.1 mV) from the isoelectric line in the standard limb leads, but a greater (ascending) S-T elevation may

normally be seen in V_{2-3}, here even
up to 3 mm.

A pathologic S-T deviation can be seen especially in strain patterns, bundle branch block, myocardial infarction, coronary insufficiency (ischemia) and after digitalis:

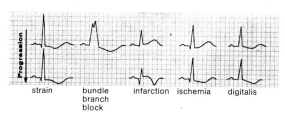

strain   bundle branch block   infarction   ischemia   digitalis

(7) T waves.

With regard to T waves, their direction is the most important feature. T waves can be

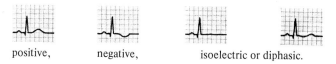

positive,   negative,   isoelectric or diphasic.

The T wave normally always is positive in leads I, II and V_{5-6} and negative in aVR. Diphasic or negative T waves are seen frequently in normal subjects in III and V_{1-2}.

Pathologically isoelectric or inverted T waves are among the most frequent abnormalities in the electrocardiogram. They occur in a large number of heart diseases, but particularly in various degrees of myocardial ischemia

as the sole electrocardiographic abnormality

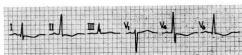

or together with S-T changes,

or as part of other characteristic patterns, as, for example,

strain and myocardial infarction.

After strongly deformed QRS complexes in, for example, ventricular extrasystoles,

bundle branch block and idioventricular rhythm,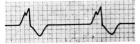

T wave changes always are found, at times called "secondary", namely secondary to the strongly altered course of the QRS deflections, and as a rule in a direction opposite to the main QRS deflection.

In addition, both S-T segment and T wave commonly are changed by a number of physiologic and pathologic factors (changes in body position, abnormalities of respiration, mental factors, drugs, etc.).

Also, the *shape of the T waves* can be characteristically altered. Most typical are

the "coronary" T waves in myocardial infarction.

The *amplitude of the T waves* is exceedingly variable in normal subjects and therefore as a rule of slight diagnostic interest. Very tall T waves can be seen, however, as a pathologic feature, particularly in

hyperpotassemia,

but the finding must be evaluated with care and repeat control electro-cardiograms are advisable.

(8) U waves.

The U wave is a flat wave following immediately after the T wave and with the same direction. In normal subjects, it is not unusual to see well-developed U waves in the

middle precordial leads V₂₋₄.

The U wave frequently is pronounced in hypopotassemia, and together with the T wave can change in a number of conditions, e.g., myocardial ischemia and cerebrovascular accidents.

(9) Q-T interval.

The Q-T interval is measured from the beginning of the QRS complex to the end of the T wave. It is the electrocardiographic measure of the duration of systole. Poorly defined T waves can make the measure-ment difficult or impossible.

The length of the Q-T interval in normal subjects varies with heart rate, and various formulae have been constructed for the relationship. One useful formula is

$$Q\text{-}T_c = \frac{Q\text{-}T}{\sqrt{R\text{-}R}}$$

where Q-T is the Q-T interval measured in the electrocardiogram, R-R is the duration of an entire cardiac cycle and $Q\text{-}T_c$, called *the corrected Q-T interval,* is the Q-T interval the patient in question must be presumed to have if his heart rate were 60 per minute. By prolonged Q-T interval is understood a $Q\text{-}T_c$ more than 0.425 second.

The Q-T interval is of particular diagnostic interest in changes in serum calcium, but the duration of systole is influenced by other factors; it can be prolonged, for example, in heart failure and can be lengthened by quinidine and shortened by digitalis.

SOME USEFUL DEFINITIONS
WITH SPECIAL REFERENCE TO
DISTURBANCES OF RHYTHM

Aberrant ventricular conduction (ventricular aberration). The pheno-menon that a supraventricular impulse arrives so early that parts of the bundle of His are refractory after the preceding beat, so that a bundle branch block pattern develops. This is a right bundle branch block pattern in 85% of the cases (as shown here).

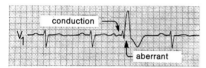

Antegrade conduction. Conduction through the atrioventricular node from atria to ventricles.

Asynchronism. A condition in which various parts of the atria or various parts of the ventricles are strongly out of phase with respect to the refractory period and conduction. Predisposes to fibrillation of the atria or ventricles.

Atrioventricular dissociation. A condition in which the atria and ventricles are activated from separate centers.

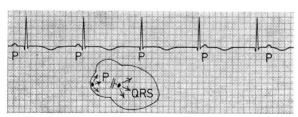

Atrioventricular junction. A modern term comprising (1) the atrio-ventricular node, (2) its transitional areas to the atria and to the bundle of His and (3) the bundle of His.

Automaticity. Spontaneous ability to emit impulses. A characteristic property of tissue in the conducting system of the heart, including the sinoatrial node, and associated with the ability of this tissue to undergo slow spontaneous diastolic depolarization (phase 4 depolarization, see textbooks).

Block. Slowed to completely interrupted conduction of an impulse in parts of the conducting system. In the widest sense, the term is used for all regions of the myocardium. A distinction often is made between (A) *functional* (physiologic) block: slowed or interrupted conduction of an impulse due to the tissue being refractory following a previous impulse, (B) *anatomic* (pathologic) block: slowed or interrupted conduction also outside the normal refractory period of the tissue.

Depending on localization, a distinction is made between sinoatrial, atrioventricular and intraventricular (most frequently bundle branch) block. According to grade, a distinction is drawn between *first degree:* slowed conduction, *second degree:* total interruption of conduction for some of the impulses and *third degree:* total interruption of conduction for all impulses.

Capture beat (capture). A conduction beat that interrupts a period with atrioventricular dissociation.

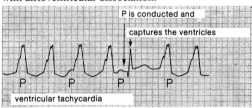

Compensatory pause. The pause after an extrasystole, "compensating" for the interval by which an extrasystole is premature ("complete compensatory pause", see sketch) or compensating partly ("incomplete compensatory pause").

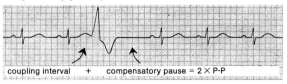

Concealed conduction. An expression often used to explain the phenomenon that conduction in the atrioventricular node is temporarily inhibited because the preceding impulse has penetrated part of the way into the node without passing through it. As the penetration cannot be seen in the electrocardiogram, the term "concealed" is used. The classic example: The beat after an interpolated ventricular extrasystole has a prolonged P-R interval, presumably because of concealed conduction of the ventricular extrasystole in a retrograde direction some distance up into the atrioventricular node.

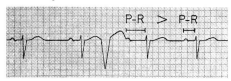

Coupling interval. The time interval between a basic rhyth beat and an extrasystole; see figure under "Compensatory pause". Not infrequently constant in the case of extrasystoles from the same focus in the same patient.

Depolarization (activation). Breakdown of the resting transmembrane potential. An impulse spreads by the depolarization of a cell "starting" the depolarization of the next. The course of the wave of depolarization in the ventricular myocardium determines the shape of the QRS complex.

Dysrhythmia. A term that is more comprehensive than arrhythmia, as logically it also includes abnormal rhythms without irregular heart action. A synonym often used is "disturbances of cardiac rhythm".

Ectopic beat. The phenomenon that an ectopic focus starts a beat in atria or ventricles or the entire heart. Comprises atrial, junctional and ventricular beats.

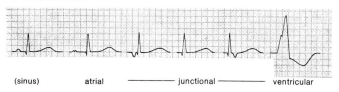

(sinus)   atrial   ———— junctional ———— ventricular

25

Ectopic focus (ectopic center). A focus other than the sinoatrial node, starting a wave of activation (depolarization).

Ectopic rhythm. The phenomenon that either the atria or the ventricles or both are activated repeatedly in sequence from an ectopic focus.

Ectopic tachycardia. A rapid rhythm, originating from an ectopic focus as a result of increased automaticity, resulting in an inherent ectopic rate of beat that is greater than the inherent rate of the sinoatrial node.

Entrance block. The phenomenon that a focus is protected in some unexplained manner against depolarization by impulses from another focus.

Escape beat. A single beat from an ectopic center, appearing after a pause in (or after slowing of) that rhythm which till then has been the leading (dominant or basic) rhythm (most often sinus rhythm).

Escape interval. The time elapsing before an escape beat or an escape rhythm appears after the start of a pause in the dominant rhythm. This interval often is longer than the interbeat interval of the inherent rhythm of the ectopic center.

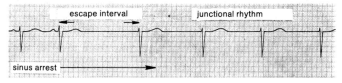

Escape rhythm. A rhythm from an ectopic center that temporarily takes over the role of the cardiac pacemaker because the hitherto leading rhythm stops or becomes slower than the intrinsic rhythm of the ectopic center.

Excitability. Tendency of an individual myocardial region to react – by depolarization – to impulses reaching it from other myocardial regions or from outside, either as mechanical impulses (e.g., from catheters) or electrical impulses (e.g., from artificial pacemakers). The excitability is abolished during the refractory period and is increased during the supernormal phase.

Exit block. The phenomenon that the impulse from an automatic focus cannot reach the surroundings. Example: sinoatrial block.

Extrasystole. An ectopic beat, arising too early ("premature beat") because of increased excitability or automaticity in an ectopic focus. See under "Re-entry" for another theory for extrasystoles as caused by a local disturbance of conduction.

Fusion beat (combination beat, summation beat). Results from simultaneous activation of the myocardium of the ventricle from two foci: *ventricular fusion beat.* A frequent characteristic is that QRS is short and of small amplitude. Originates most often by a sinus rhythm impulse and an ectopic ventricular impulse reaching the ventricles simultaneously.

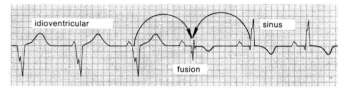

Atrial fusion beat occurs in an analogous manner by simultaneous activation of the atria from two foci, but often is more difficult to diagnose. The QRS complexes in the W-P-W syndrome are a special form of ventricular fusion beats. Here, however, the time difference results in broad complexes.

Idiojunctional rhythm (old term: idionodal rhythm). Ectopic junctional rhythm that controls only the ventricles.

Idioventricular rhythm. Ectopic ventricular rhythm that controls only the ventricles.

Interference. Used with different meanings in the textbooks. The classic significance of the word (as used here) means the phenomenon in which sinus impulses singly or in series are conducted during atrioventricular

27

dissociation and thus temporarily cancel this dissociation ("interfere with this dissociation"). The conducted beats are called ventricular capture beats.

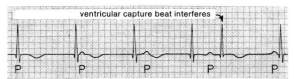

Junctional beats and rhythms (= atrioventricular [AV] junctional beats and rhythms). Ectopic beats and rhythms from a focus in the atrioventricular junction (see p. 23). The term now is commonly used instead of "nodal" and "atrioventricular [AV] nodal" beats and rhythms. Experimental studies have shown that there are no automatic fibers in the atrioventricular node itself. Junctional ectopic centers therefore are extranodal. In this atlas, the term "nodal" accordingly is preserved only for conduction disturbances.

Nodal (= atrioventricular [AV] nodal). See "Junctional beats and rhythms".

Parasystole. The phenomenon that an ectopic focus maintains its automaticity independent of and simultaneously with the sinoatrial node. The two foci compete on an equal basis. Presupposes the theory of entrance block.

Premature beat = extrasystole.

Re-entry. The phenomenon that, after having activated a region, the same impulse again activates this after having traveled over a path within another region. The phenomenon explains reciprocal beats; see page 117. According to one theory, the phenomenon also explains ventricular extrasystoles by assuming unidirectional block in a localized myocardial area, resulting in re-entry (②) of the original normal sinus impulse (①) after delay in the area peripheral to the unidirectional block; see sketch. This theory, explaining the extrasystole as a disturbance of conduction, is not generally accepted or supported by experimental data; see, therefore, under definition of extrasystole.

28

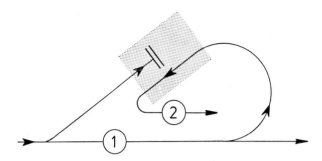

Refractory period. The time interval in which the excitability of *the single myocardial cell* is abolished (absolute refractory period) or reduced (relative refractory period). Followed by a short interval with increased excitability (supernormal phase). For the *myocardium as a whole*, there are no sharp boundaries for these periods, because of the time differences between the membrane potentials of the individual cells.

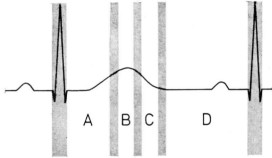

Generally speaking, *the ventricles as a whole are absolutely refractory* from the end of QRS to slightly into the T wave (A). In a period around the peak of the T wave, some regions still are absolutely refractory, some are relatively refractory and some are not refractory. In this phase, it will be especially easy for a single electrical impulse to release electrical chaos, resulting in fibrillation. This is therefore called *the vulnerable phase* (B). *The supernormal phase* (C) may, in practice, be recognized by the fact that in this period artificial pacemaker impulses have a lower threshold value than in the nonrefractory period (D).

Repolarization. Rebuilding of the membrane potential. It is a restitution phenomenon and not a propagated phenomenon (converse to depolarization). The temporal differences in the repolarization of different regions of the myocardium determine the placing, width, direction and shape of the S-T segment and the T wave.

Retrograde conduction. Conduction through the atrioventricular node in the direction from ventricles to atria. More universally used for propagation of an impulse in a direction opposite to that of normal.

Supernormal excitability is present in the supernormal phase, corresponding to the last part of the T wave and the U wave; see under "Refractory period".

Supraventricular beats and rhythms. Term used when it cannot be seen from the electrocardiogram whether the beat or the rhythm comes from the sinoatrial node, the atria or the atrioventricular junction.

Unidirectional block. Impulses can be led in one direction but not in the opposite direction. The term most often describes conduction in the atrioventricular node, where the block usually is retrograde, whereas antegrade conduction is possible.

Vulnerable phase. The phase around the peak of the T wave, where a single electrical impulse most easily triggers off fibrillation; see under "Refractory period".

CHARACTERISTIC
ELECTROCARDIOGRAMS

An asterisk after a figure number indicates that the example is less important for beginners and for personnel at a basic training level.

1

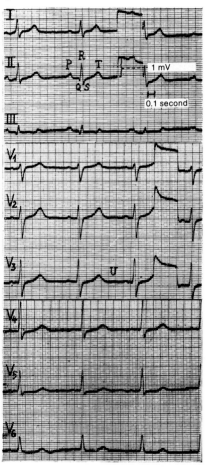

THE NORMAL 9-LEAD ELECTROCARDIOGRAM

Extremity leads

I – II – III

= Einthoven's standard limb leads, where the wires are so connected to the electrocardiograph that at any moment

II = I + III

I = left arm – right arm
II = left leg – right arm
III = left leg – left arm

Normal values (simplified)

	$P < 0.12$ second
	P-R (or P-Q) ≤ 0.22 second
	$QRS < 0.12$ second
	$P \leq 2\frac{1}{2}$ mm
I-III	$Q \leq 3$ mm
	$R <$ about 25 mm
	$S <$ about 8 mm
	T_I and T_{II} = 1-7 mm
	T_{III} varying (pos. or neg.)
	Q-T$_c$ ≤ 0.425

Precordial leads

V$_1$ – V$_2$ – V$_3$ – V$_4$ – V$_5$ – V$_6$.

V = precordium – reference electrode ('Wilson's central terminal electrode")

Precordial electrodes are placed as follows:

V$_1$: 4th right intercostal space near sternum

V$_2$: 4th left intercostal space near sternum

V$_3$: Midway between V$_2$ and V$_4$

V$_4$: 5th left intercostal space in the mid-clavicular line

V$_5$: Left anterior axillary line at the same horizontal level as V$_4$

V$_6$: Left midaxillary line at the same horizontal level as V$_4$

P: often negative in V$_{1-2}$, rarely negative in V$_{3-4}$, never negative in V$_{5-6}$

QRS: rS pattern in V$_{1-2}$, RS pattern in V$_{3-4}$, qRs pattern in V$_{5-6}$, (q and s may be missing)

V$_1$-V$_6$

S-T segment: often elevated in V$_{1-4}$

T: often negative in V$_{1-2}$, more rarely negative in V$_3$, never (in adults) negative in V$_{4-6}$

3

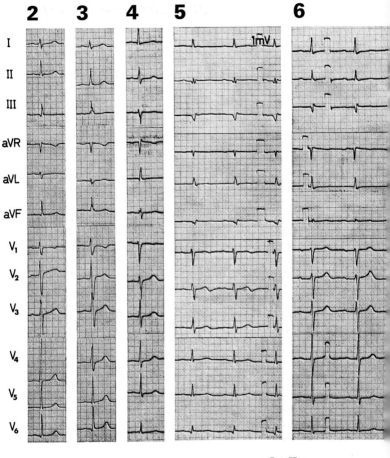

$$\text{Lead from right arm aVR} = -\left(\frac{\text{I} + \text{II}}{2}\right)$$

$$\text{Lead from left arm aVL} = \frac{\text{I} - \text{III}}{2}$$

$$\text{Lead from left leg aVF} = \frac{\text{II} + \text{III}}{2}$$

UNIPOLAR EXTREMITY LEADS

The unipolar extremity leads aVR, aVL and aVF are recorded in many places as routine. They may be regarded as a supplementary way of reading the electrocardiogram, even though they do not contain information not already included in three *simultaneously recorded* standard limb leads. At any moment of the cardiac cycle, there are in fact simple relationships that hold; see page 34. aVR, aVL and aVF are easily recorded with all the electrocardiographs on the market. Normally, aVR will be dominated by negative deflections in P, QRS and T whereas aVL and aVF will vary more. In axis shifts as a consequence of changes in position of the heart or ventricular hypertrophy, aVR, aVL and aVF will change simultaneously with I, II and III, in agreement with the formulae on page 34.

It is generally considered that in certain diseases unipolar leads give a clearer – more easily readable or more logical – picture than that obtained simply by I, II and III. As an example of this might be mentioned that the significance of a Q_{III} for the diagnosis of inferior myocardial infarction is uncertain, whereas a large Q wave in aVF is more direct evidence of inferior infarction.

Whether these leads should be employed in the daily routine in all cases is more or less a matter of individual choice. They do not provide any real increase in the diagnostic information. In any case, I, II and III are always recorded at the same time.

2-4 **Examples of normal unipolar extremity leads:** *aVF is an "intermediate between II and III,"* and *aVR is a "mirror image of an intermediate between I and II";* cf. the formulae opposite. Normally therefore, aVR will be dominated by negative deflections whereas aVL and aVF alter with the electrical axis. In pronounced (pathologic) cases, aVR also changes with the axis; see pages 42-43.

5 **Q wave in aVF.** Patient with inferolateral myocardial infarction. A well-pronounced (wide and notched) *Q wave* is seen *in aVF.* For comparison:

6 **Patient with normal heart and obesity.** There is admittedly a large Q_{III} but no Q wave in aVF (which merely expresses the fact that simultaneously with Q in lead III there is a positive deflection in lead II; cf. formula for aVF).

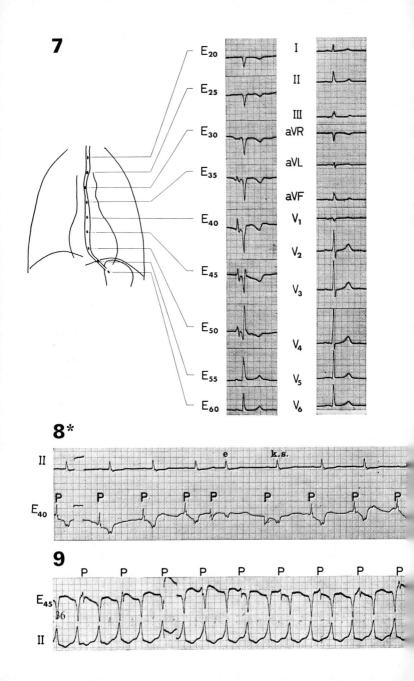

7

E₂₀
E₂₅
E₃₀
E₃₅
E₄₀
E₄₅
E₅₀
E₅₅
E₆₀

I
II
III
aVR
aVL
aVF
V₁
V₂
V₃
V₄
V₅
V₆

8*

II

E₄₀   P   P   P   P   P   P   P   P   P

e   k.s.

9   P   P   P   P   P   P   P   P   P

E₄₅
36
II

ESOPHAGEAL LEADS

In esophageal leads, the one electrode is placed in the esophagus while the other electrode is Wilson's central terminal electrode. These leads are designated E_{25}-E_{35}, etc., where E signifies esophageal lead and the number indicates the distance (in cm) of the electrode from the nares.

The esophageal leads have been used to assist in diagnosis of *inferior myocardial infarction.* This use, however, involves important sources of error: it is necessary to ensure that the electrode is right down behind the ventricles, since in leads behind the atria and higher up. there are *normally large Q waves.* The form of the P waves can give an indication of the placing of the electrodes.

These leads are better suited to *elucidate dysrhythmias,* as the P waves become especially clear in the leads just behind the atria. (Intracardial leads are also excellent for this purpose.)

7   Normal esophageal leads. When the electrode is cranial to the heart (E_{20}-E_{30}), the *P waves* are low and inverted. In the vicinity of the atria (E_{40}-E_{50}), the P waves are tall, peaked and diphasic. When the electrode is in the vicinity of the ventricles (E_{55}-E_{60}), the P waves are low and positive. A position with high P waves (E_{40}-E_{45}) is suitable to evaluate dysrhythmias. The *QRS complex* normally shows conspicuous Q waves or QS waves in the leads at or cranial to the atrioventricular boundary (E_{20}-E_{50}), and the *T waves* usually are negative in the same leads. To evaluate inferior infarction in this patient it would be necessary to go right down to E_{55}-E_{60}.

8   Arrhythmia elucidated by esophageal lead. The P waves are not very pronounced in lead II. Lead E_{40} shows that the extrasystole (e) is atrial, as it has a P wave of a shape other than those of the sinus beats and with a longer P-R interval. It is further seen that also the compensatory beat (k.S.) is ectopic, as the shape of the P wave is deviant.

9   Lead II suggests ventricular tachycardia, but it could be a case of supraventricular tachycardia with aberrant ventricular conduction, or in a patient with bundle branch block. The esophageal lead (E_{45}) clearly shows the slower P rhythm (atrioventricular dissociation), i.e., **ventricular tachycardia** is present; cf. page 103.

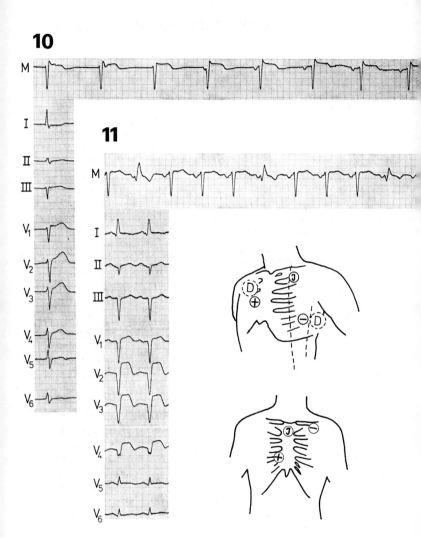

MONITORING LEADS (M LEADS)

In electrocardiographic monitoring in coronary units and other intensive care wards, artifacts can be reduced by avoiding electrodes on the extremities. *A bipolar precordial lead* (*"monitor lead," "modified chest electrode"* and other designations) is therefore used. The term *"monitoring lead"* is used in the present atlas, abbreviated to *M lead or merely M*. It is an advantage for the evaluation if the M lead resembles V_1. As a rule, this will give clear P waves and also allows evaluation of the patterns in bundle branch block configuration and ectopic ventricular beats. The sketches on page 38 show two ways of doing this. The upper sketch is used with M leads in this book and does not give quite so clean a V_1 as with the lower arrangement. $\oplus$ and $\ominus$ are the different electrodes. $\textcircled{J}$ signifies earth. $\textcircled{D}$ signifies electrode placing during defibrillation if necessary. The precordium is also accessible for auscultation.

NB: remember that normally the P waves (with antegrade conduction) often are negative in the M lead, particularly with electrode placing as in the upper sketch.

10 **Arrhythmia diagnostics in M lead.** The monitoring M lead clearly shows P waves, and the QRS complexes have a reasonably good resemblance to those in V_1 (cf. V_1 with the first beat in M). The M lead shows junctional rhythm with atrioventricular dissociation (the first five beats), changing to sinus rhythm (the last three beats). Cf. also **132,** page 111.

11 **Complexes with right bundle branch block pattern in M lead.** The figure shows that the M lead is an imitation of V_1. It can therefore be seen immediately that the abnormal beats (2^d, 6th and 10th complex) have a configuration like that of right bundle branch block (cf. p. 51) and appear after normal P waves. This, therefore, probably is a case of sinus beats with aberrant ventricular conduction, as such in fact often give right bundle branch block pattern. Patient with acute anteroseptal-anteroapical myocardial infarction (cf. p. 67) and possibly LAH (left anterior hemiblock; cf. p. 55).

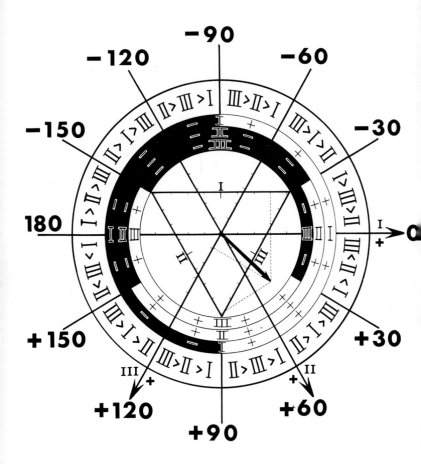

12 Figure for evaluation of the QRS axis. The signs of the net areas
of the three standard limb leads determine the placing of the axis
within 60° sectors (the black-white three inner circles), while a more
accurate placing within 30° sectors then is determined from the relative
mutual sizes of the three net areas (outer circle).

ELECTRICAL AXIS OF THE HEART

By the electrical axis of the heart is understood in general the average axis for the QRS complex. This is determined by examining the areas in the standard limb leads, reckoned with sign, and called for simplicity "the net area" of QRS. For example:

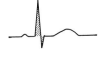 Positive net area of QRS, the hatched area above the isoelectric line being greater than the hatched area below the line.

 Negative net area of QRS, the downwardly directed hatched area being greater than the sum of the two upwardly directed areas.

I

III

 Positive net area in lead I, negative in lead III. In addition, it is easily seen that III > I, i.e., the net area in lead III is *numerically* greater than that in lead I.

By a simple area evaluation like the above, the mean QRS axis can be easily determined within a 30° range with the aid of a figure as, e.g., **12.**

Normal axis is a mean QRS axis in the region from 0° to + 90°.

Right axis deviation: from +90° through 180° to −90°.

Left axis deviation: from 0° to −90°.

Figure **12** can also explain the rules for axis deviation, which follow on page 43.

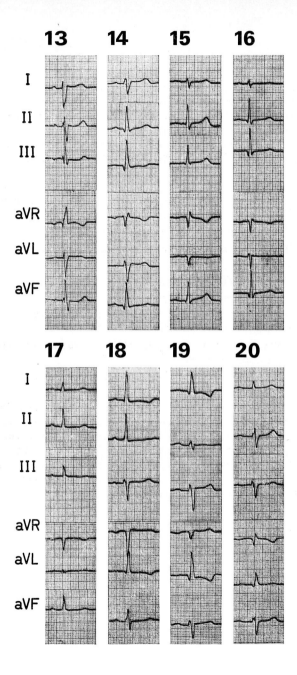

The following simple rules are valid for the *QRS complexes:*

(1) *Right axis deviation* is present when in lead I there is a greater area under the isoelectric line than above (negative net area), *no matter how the other leads appear.*

(2) *Left axis deviation* is present when the net area in lead I is positive and in lead III is negative, *provided that* the net area in III is not the least of the areas in the three extremity leads I, II and III.

13 **Pronounced right axis deviation:** the net area in lead I is strongly negative and, in addition, the area in II is negative.

14 **Right axis deviation:** the net area in lead I is negative.

15 **Slight right axis deviation:** slightly negative net area of QRS in lead I.

16 **Normal axis** (all net areas positive).

17 **Normal axis** (all net areas positive).

18 **Normal axis:** Admittedly, the net area in lead III is negative, but it is numerically less than that of lead I and that of lead II.

19 **Left axis deviation:** net area in lead III negative and not the least of the areas in the three leads.

20 **Pronounced left axis deviation:** negative net area in both leads III and II.

The figures show the corresponding *configuration of the unipolar limb leads* aVR, aVL and aVF. Note that *aVR varies least:* it is dominated by negative deflections, except in pronounced right axis deviation. Further, as a *main* rule, aVL has a dominating R wave in left axis deviation and in the most horizontal normal axes whereas aVF has a dominating R wave in (non-extreme) right axis deviation and in the most vertical normal axes. Cf. page 35.

21

I

II   1 mVolt

III

V₁

V₂

V₃

V₄

V₅

V₆

22

I

II

III

V₁

V₂

V₃

V₄

V₅

V₆

23

I

II

III

V₁

V₂

V₃

V₄

V₅

V₆

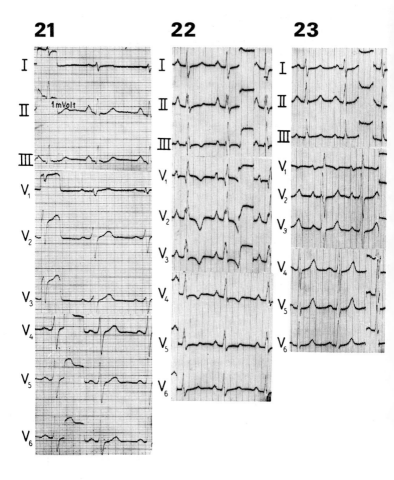

ATRIAL ENLARGEMENT

The reliability of the electrocardiographic diagnosis of atrial enlargement is limited. Abnormal P waves may occur in healthy subjects or in intra-atrial conduction disturbances, and atrial enlargement may be present without P wave abnormalities. With this in mind, the rules are the following:

(1) In *enlargement or hypertrophy of the right atrium,* the P waves, especially in leads II and III, are high (> 0.25 mV), peaked and of normal duration ($\leqq 0.10$ second). The P waves in the right precordial leads are positive/negative diphasic with a high positive component.

(2) In *enlargement or hypertrophy of the left atrium,* the P waves, especially in leads I and II, are wide (> 0.10 second) and notched. Notching ("two-humped" P waves) is most important if the P waves are wide and/or high. The P waves in the right precordial leads are positive/negative diphasic with a deep and wide negative component.

Finally, it should be recalled that atrial enlargement involves a disposition to atrial fibrillation and flutter.

21 Patient with chronic pulmonary disease. There are signs of **enlargement of the right atrium** in the form of tall and peaked P waves in leads II and III ("P pulmonale"), no P changes in the other leads. In addition, there is right axis deviation and rS or RS pattern in all precordial leads; cf. page 47.

22 Patient with congenital pulmonary stenosis. There are signs of **enlargement of the right atrium** in the form af tall and peaked P waves in leads I and II. Diphasic P wave in V_1 with high positive component. High and peaked P in V_{2-3}. In addition, there is right axis deviation and in the precordial leads signs of right ventricular hypertrophy and strain; cf. page 49.

23 Patient with mitral stenosis. There are signs of **enlargement of the left atrium** in the form of P waves increased in width in leads I and II, two-humped in lead I ("P mitrale"). In addition, there is an increase in the amplitude of P_{II} and diphasic P in V_1 with equal positive and negative components. The precordial leads show signs of right ventricular hypertrophy without strain; cf. page 47.

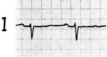
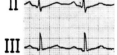
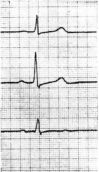

I

II

III

V₁

V₂

V₃

V₄

V₅

V₆

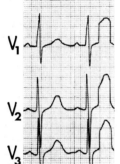
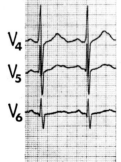
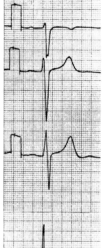
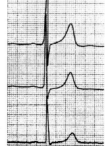

VENTRICULAR HYPERTROPHY

Axis deviation can be due to abnormal position of the heart, unilateral ventricular hypertrophy or bundle branch block. In addition, an abnormal mean QRS axis may result from patterns of myocardial infarction, pre-excitation and ectopic rhythms.

Ventricular hypertrophy is diagnosed mainly from the precordial leads, where the main feature is the finding of large R waves in leads facing the hypertrophic ventricle and large S waves in the contralateral leads.

Hypertrophy of the right ventricle results in high R waves in V_1 and conspicuous S waves in V_{5-6}. Lead V_1 may have a qR, qRs, R, Rs or RS pattern or a notched or double R wave (RsR'). Conventional criteria for hypertrophy are an R/S ratio $\geqq 1.0$ and – provided that V_1 lacks a q wave – an amplitude of the R wave of at least 0.7 mV. A diagnosis of right ventricular hypertrophy is supported by the finding of right axis deviation and/or right ventricular strain (see p. 49). It may be added that also an electrocardiogram with an rS pattern in all precordial leads is said to be suggestive of right ventricular enlargement.

Hypertrophy of the left ventricle results in high R waves in V_{5-6} and deep S waves in V_{1-2}. Numerous voltage criteria for the diagnosis of left ventricular hypertrophy are advanced, e.g., that the sum of the amplitude of S in V_1 or V_2 and R in V_5 or V_6 is greater than 3.5 mV. A diagnosis of left ventricular hypertrophy is supported by one or more of the following: left ventricular strain (p. 49), left axis deviation, signs of left atrial enlargement and a delayed intrinsicoid deflection in V_{5-6} (the interval from the beginning of QRS to the peak of the R wave $\geqq 0.05$ second). Some authors try to increase the diagnostic validity by including these features in a point score system (see textbooks).

Combined hypertrophy (left + right) is a very difficult electrocardiographic diagnosis to establish.

24 **Hypertrophy of the right ventricle.** Ratio R/S in V_1 is about 1.7 with an R amplitude of 1.6 mV, and S waves are conspicuous right out in V_{5-6}. In addition, the standard limb leads show right axis deviation.

25 **Probable hypertrophy of the left ventricle.** There are very tall R waves over the left ventricle, S in V_2 + R in V_5 = 6.0 mV. Other criteria for left ventricular hypertrophy are absent.

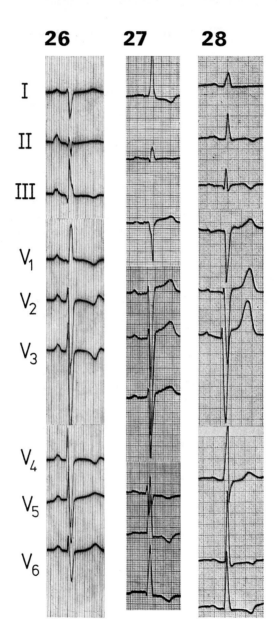

ELECTROCARDIOGRAPHIC STRAIN PATTERN

In severe and prolonged hypertrophy of a ventricle, characteristic changes in the S-T segments and T waves often appear in addition to the QRS changes (p. 47). In leads over the hypertrophic ventricle, i.e., those leads characterized by tall R waves, a *depressed S-T segment* appears *with flattened or negative/positive diphasic or completely inverted T waves.* This pattern often is called "strain pattern". In addition to supporting the diagnosis of hypertrophy, the strain pattern probably can be taken as evidence for a certain degree of myocardial ischemia in the hypertrophic ventricle.

Right ventricular strain is seen in the right precordial leads and III, possibly II. Left ventricular strain is seen in the left precordial leads and I, possibly II. It must be remembered, however, that young subjects with left ventricular hypertrophy and vertical position of the heart may have *left* ventricular strain patterns in the standard leads III and II instead of I and II.

26 **Right ventricular strain.** Right axis deviation is seen together with hypertrophy of the right ventricle. The strain pattern appears in the form of negative T in III and V_1 as well as diphasic T in V_{2-4} with slight S-T depression in the last leads.

27 **Left ventricular strain.** Left axis deviation is seen together with hypertrophy of the left ventricle. The strain pattern appears in the form of S-T depression with inverted T waves in I and V_{4-6}.

28 **Vertical heart and left ventricular strain.** Young woman with left ventricular hypertrophy (deep S in V_{1-3} and tall R in V_{5-6}). As the heart is vertical, the axis here is normal. The strain pattern presents as a depression of S-T with inverted T wave in V_{5-6}. In the standard limb leads, the inversion is most pronounced in III and II.

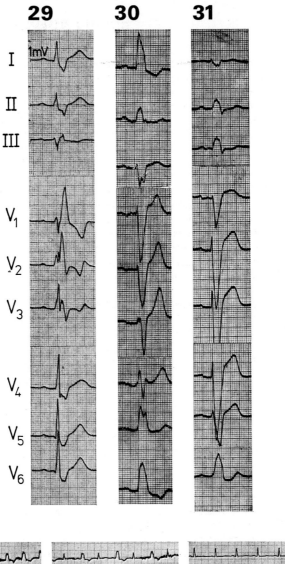

29

I

II

III

V₁

V₂

V₃

V₄

V₅

V₆

30

31

1mV

32

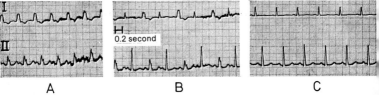

I

II

H
0.2 second

A   B   C

BUNDLE BRANCH BLOCK

The term bundle branch block is used when the duration of the QRS complex in conducted beats is at least 0.12 second.

Side localization is seen from the precordial leads.

Right bundle branch block is characterized by a double R wave (M-shape) or a large, wide, possibly notched R wave in V_{1-2} and a wide S wave in V_{5-6}.

Left bundle branch block is characterized by a wide, deep S wave (and a small or missing R wave) in V_{1-2} and a wide, large R wave in V_6 or V_{5-6}.

The following figures illustrate that the side localization is easily seen in the precordial leads. As a rule, it is enough to examine V_1.

In bundle branch block it is the rule that the main deflection of the S-T segment + T wave is in the opposite direction to the main deflection in QRS. As a rule, therefore, there is a depressed S-T segment and a negative T wave in leads with tall, wide R waves. As a result, the S-T + T configuration resembles strain patterns.

29 Typical right bundle branch block. The duration of QRS is 0.17 second (V_{1-3}), and there are M-shaped complexes in V_1. Note that the S-T segments and T waves resemble those in right ventricular strain.

30 Typical left bundle branch block. The duration of QRS is 0.14 second (V_1), and there are wide, deep S waves and quite small R waves in V_{1-2}. Note that the S-T segments and T waves resemble those in left ventricular strain.

31 Left bundle branch block. The duration of QRS is 0.14 second. Deep, broad S waves in V_{1-2}. As a rule, the electrical axis in bundle branch block follows the side localization, but here there is right axis deviation in the standard leads I-III, which, in addition, show small deflections, earlier often called "arborization block."

32 Intermittent bundle branch block. (A) Bundle branch block, probably left (missing precordial leads), in a 64-year-old woman. (B) High oxygen breathing during anesthesia. Now only every second beat shows bundle branch block. (C) Under continued high oxygen percentage in the inspired air, the bundle branch block disappears.

Intermittent bundle branch block probably is a transitional stage to permanent bundle branch block.

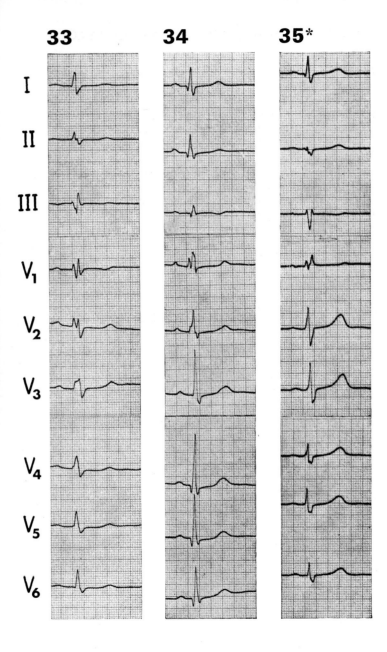

	33	34	35*
I			
II			
III			
V₁			
V₂			
V₃			
V₄			
V₅			
V₆			

INCOMPLETE RIGHT BUNDLE BRANCH BLOCK

The term incomplete right bundle branch block usually is applied to an electrocardiogram where the QRS configuration is as in right bundle branch block, but where the duration of QRS is from 0.08 to 0.11 second. The most characteristic feature is that the leads over the right ventricle, especially V_1, show two R waves, the latter being the larger. In addition, there often is a rather wide S wave in the left precordial leads.

Incomplete right bundle branch block is not uncommonly found as a normal variant, but, in addition, it is a characteristic finding in atrial septal defect and in certain cases of chronic cor pulmonale, and it can have a transient appearance in pulmonary embolism.

Three patients with incomplete right bundle branch block:

33 QRS duration 0.10 second. V_1 shows an rSR's' pattern.

34 QRS duration 0.09 second. V_1 shows an rsR's' pattern.

35 QRS duration 0.08 second. Also this patient has double R wave in V_1, namely an rsR' pattern. The standard leads show slight left axis deviation, presumably an expression of a simultaneous LAH (see p. 55 for this). This combination is characteristic of *primum* defect in the atrial septum.

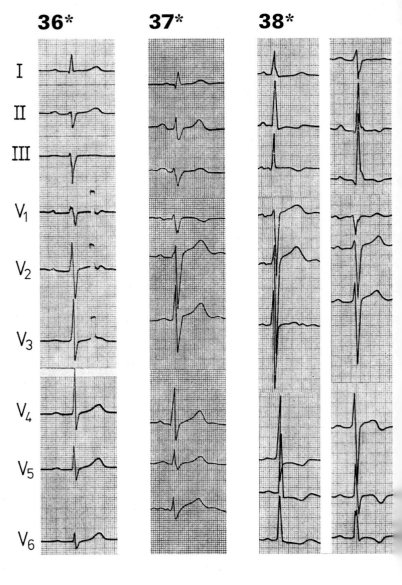

36*   37*   38*

I
II
III
V₁
V₂
V₃
V₄
V₅
V₆

54

A   B

LEFT HEMIBLOCKS

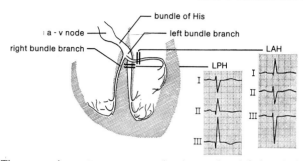

There now is greater agreement that incomplete left bundle branch blocks often can be diagnosed. More or less clearly, the left branch of the bundle of His can be distinguished as a thin anterior and a thick posterior branch. *LAH ("left anterior hemiblock")* is characterized by a small initial q in I simultaneously with a small, narrow r in II and III, followed by a main deflection in QRS with an axis around −60°, i.e., a wide, tall R in I and a wide, deep S in II and III (see **12,** p. 40). QRS duration is less than 0.12 second. Pure *LPH ("left posterior hemiblock")* is difficult to diagnose. The diagnosis is very probable if QRS is less than 0.12 second, there is a narrow initial r in I simultaneously with a small q in II and III, followed by a main deflection in QRS with an axis about +120°, i.e., a wide and deep S in I and a tall, wide R in II and III (see **12,** p. 40), but only provided that this pattern is not merely due to right ventricular hypertrophy or vertical position of the heart. The latter can be very difficult to demonstrate.

36 LAH. Note the initial q in I and r in II and III, while the main axis of QRS is about −60° (positive deflection in I, negative in II and III, and the area in I is approx. = II). Ten-year-old girl with primum defect in the atrial septum.

37 LAH. Same features as in **36.** QRS wider, but < 12 seconds.

38 LPH. (A) Boy aged 11 years with aortic stenosis. Left ventricular hypertrophy with strain and normal axis. (B) Aged 17 years, 6 years after aortic valvulotomy. Now initial r in I and q in II and III, while the main axis of QRS is approx. +110° (see **12,** p. 40). As this patient continues to have some aortic disease, it is not merely vertical position of the heart; in other words, an LPH has developed.

39*

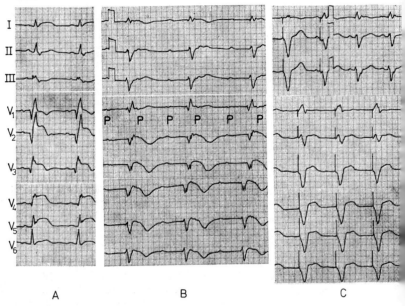

I II III V$_1$ V$_2$ V$_3$ V$_4$ V$_5$ V$_6$

P P P P P P

A   B   C

40*

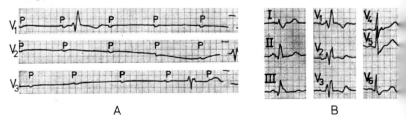

V$_1$ V$_2$ V$_3$

P P P P P

I II III V$_1$ V$_2$ V$_3$ V$_4$ V$_5$ V$_6$

A   B

BILATERAL BUNDLE BRANCH BLOCK

By *bifascicular (bilateral) bundle branch block* is understood simultaneous block in the right branch of the bundle of His and in one of the left branches (figure, p. 55). If the remaining bundle branch is also blocked, we then have a *complete trifascicular block,* which cannot be distinguished electrocardiographically from other third degree atrioventricular block (see p. 125). If there is only incomplete block in the remaining branch, then we obtain a bifascicular block pattern + first degree or second degree atrioventricular block, i.e., *trifascicular block that can be diagnosed.*

Patients with bilateral bundle branch block are to some degree likely to develop third degree atrioventricular block with Adams-Stokes attacks, and prophylactic treatment with an artificial pacemaker is recommended by some authors.

39 **Right bundle branch block + left anterior hemiblock (LAH) + partial 2:1 atrioventricular block = trifascicular block.** (A) 42-year-old man with right bundle branch block (wide QRS and double R wave in V_1) and acute anterior infarction (pronounced elevations of S-T in I and V_{2-6} and Q waves in V_{1-4}). (B) Two days later, right bundle branch block still is seen (V_1), but the QRS configuration in I-III has changed and now satisfies the criteria for LAH (see p. 55). At the same time there is 2:1 atrioventricular block. As trifascicular block thus is present, pacemaker treatment is instituted: (C) Constant artificial pacemaker rhythm in V_{1-6}. In leads I-III the first beat is triggered off by the pacemaker, beats 3 and 4 are sinus beats with such a high rate that the demand pacemaker is inhibited, beat no. 2 is a fusion beat (cf. p. 27). The pure sinus beats still show right bundle branch block + LAH, but now the P-R conduction is normal.

40 **Right bundle branch block + left posterior hemiblock (LPH).** Patient with Adams-Stokes attack. (A) During a pre-attack state, third degree atrioventricular block is recorded with very slow ventricular rate (V_{1-3} have not been recorded simultaneously). (B) In a period without attacks, right bundle branch block is seen (double R in V_1) while at the same time I-III suggest LPH: Initial small r in I and q in II and III, while the wide, last part of QRS has S in I and large R in II and III; cf. the criteria, page 55.

41

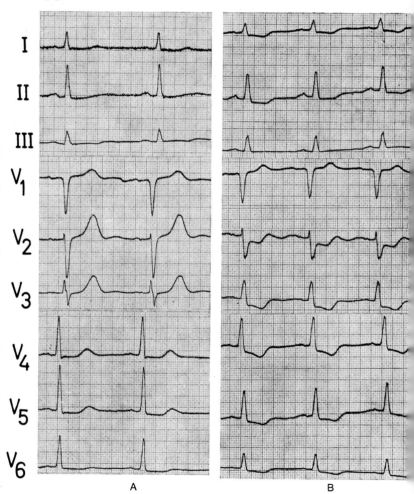

I

II

III

V₁

V₂

V₃

V₄

V₅

V₆

A   B

Coronary insufficiency is the most common cause of myocardial ischemia. The most frequent and most important electrocardiographic signs of myocardial ischemia are as follows:

(1) *Flat depression of the S-T segment, or depression with slope downward to the right, in several leads,*

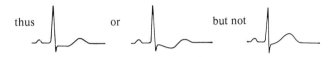

(2) *Isoelectric, diphasic or inverted T waves* in several leads other than III, V_1 and V_2 (where the T inversion is a normal phenomenon).

When changes in the electrocardiogram of the types mentioned here are only slightly pronounced, it often is difficult to decide whether they are due to myocardial ischemia or have some other cause. In that case, it may be of assistance to record the electrocardiogram (a) during attacks of chest pain or (b) before and after load with physical work ("exercise test", see pp. 63-65).

41 **Angina pectoris.** (A) Electrocardiogram from a middle-aged man with a history suggesting angina pectoris. The slight S-T depression in II, III and V_{4-6} with flat T wave in II, III and V_6 arouses a suspicion of coronary insuffiency. (B) was recorded during a spontaneous attack of angina pectoris and clearly shows myocardial ischemia in the form of depression of S-T with flattening of T in several leads (I, II and V_{2-6}).

42

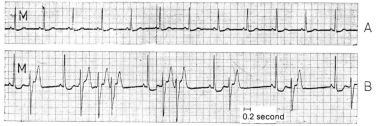

A

B

0.2 second

43*

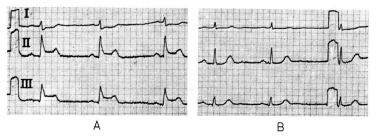

A

B

44*

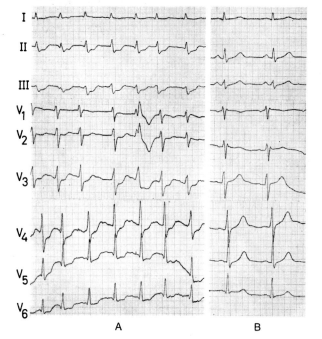

A

B

CORONARY INSUFFICIENCY 2

42 In electrocardiographic **monitoring of patients with a view to verifying the diagnosis angina pectoris,** it is an advantage to use an M lead resembling V_{5-6}, for example, by putting ⊕ lateral to the ictus and ⊖ under the left clavicle (cf sketches, p. 38). The upper curve (A) shows a recording with such a lead just before a spontaneous attack of precordial pain. During the pain attack (B), a flat depression of the S-T segment is seen and, in addition, multifocal ventricular extrasystoles.

43 **Paradoxical change in S-T during angina pectoris** ("variant angina"). In this 66-year-old woman with repeated attacks of angina pectoris at rest during days without any clinical or enzymatic signs of infarction (*"unstable angina," " preinfarction angina"*), pronounced *elevation* of S-T was seen in II and III during the attacks (A); this elevation disappeared (B) together with the pain in the course of a few minutes. The changes closely resemble the most acute phase of inferior infarction; see page 67, upper sketch.

44 **Carbon monoxide poisoning.** Also in subjects with normal coronary vessels, electrocardiographic signs of myocardial ischemia can be seen, namely in severe generalized hypoxia, e.g., in carbon monoxide poisoning and in acute *severe* respiratory insufficiency. (A) The electrocardiogram from a 35-year-old man who is unconscious from carbon monoxide poisoning. In addition to the depressions of S-T, especially in II, III and V_{3-6}, a slight increase in width of QRS complexes, atrial fibrillation with rapid ventricular response and a ventricular extrasystole (fifth beat in V_{1-3}) are seen. The next day (B), the electrocardiogram is normal (there is a double R wave in V_{1-2}, but r′ is smaller than r and S wave is so deep that it must be regarded as normal: rSr′ pattern; cf., in addition, p. 53).

(The fifth beat in V_{1-3} in curve [A] may also be an aberrant conducted beat; cf. **92,** p. 95).

45

46

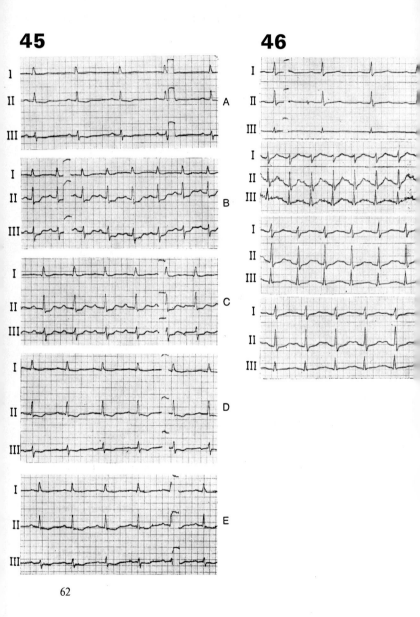

CORONARY INSUFFICIENCY
EXERCISE TEST 1

The electrocardiogram is recorded at intervals of minutes after exercise. If technically possible, recordings during the exercise will yield additional information. The type of exercise (step test, bicycle ergometry, etc.) is of little importance. The patient should be carefully supervised. Signs of a positive exercise test, indicative of coronary insufficiency (myocardial ischemia), are: (1) S-T depression of a shape as mentioned on page 59. (2) Diphasic or inverted T wave in one or more of leads I, II, V$_{4-6}$. (3) Bundle branch block. (4) Ventricular extrasystoles. (5) Disturbances of atrioventricular conduction (block). (6) Angina pectoris with immediate response to nitrates.

45 **Positive exercise test.** Woman, 52 years old, admitted for suspected coronary heart disease. (A) Slight S-T depression with diphasic T wave in II and III. Immediately following exercise (B), the electrocardiogram reveals a pronounced plane depression of S-T$_{II-III}$, which is rapidly regressing but still present 8 minutes after exercise (E). A plane S-T depression of such a magnitude allows a diagnosis of coronary insufficiency. Furthermore, the electrocardiogram 2 minutes after exercise (C) shows an increase of the P-R interval.

46 **Negative exercise test.** Low limits for abnormality of S-T depression (as low as 0.5 mm = 0.05 mV is used in some clinics) result in many false positive responses. A more reasonable limit of 1.0 or 1.5 mm (= 0.1 or 0.15 mV) will of course give some false negative responses. Of even more importance is the shape of the S-T segment (see p. 59) and problems of definition of the isoelectric baseline. In pronounced tachycardia after exercise, the interval from the T wave to the next P wave (T-P interval) is ill defined and, if so, isoelectricity is defined by the final level of the P-R interval. (A) Normal standard limb leads in a middle-aged man with atypical precordial pain without response to nitrates. Immediately after exercise, the recording (B) shows axis shift to the right and tachycardia with S-T depression; *but* the shape of the S-T segment is upward sloping, the T-P interval is ill defined and the S-T segment is starting only insignificantly below the final P-R level. The changes gradually disappear 4 (C) and 8 (D) minutes after exercise. Conclusion: Not indicative of coronary insufficiency.

47

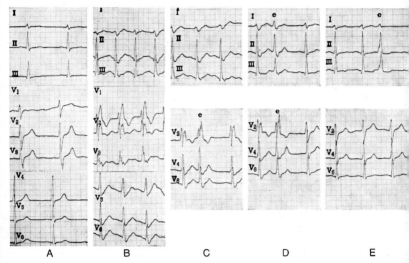

A   B   C   D   E

48*

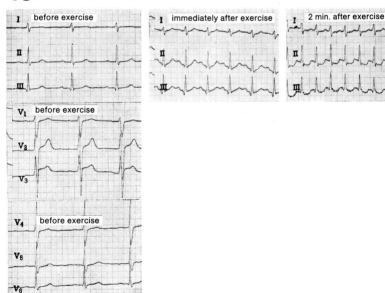

A   B   C

47 **Suggestively positive exercise test.** Middle-aged man with palpitation and dyspnea on effort. At rest (A), a normal electrocardiogram. Immediately after exercise (B), the standard limb leads show a fluctuation between normal QRS and bundle branch block, whereas the precordial leads have right bundle branch block in all beats. Two minutes after exercise (C) there still is right bundle branch block and an extrasystole (e). Also 4 minutes (D) and 8 minutes (E) after exercise, extrasystoles (e) are seen, whereas the bundle branch block disappears gradually.

48 **"False positive" exercise test.** Younger man, complaining of palpitation after effort. Rest electrocardiogram (A) is normal. Immediately after exercise (B), no pathologic exercise reaction is seen; cf. text to **46,** page 63. Two minutes after exercise (C), the electrocardiogram shows tachycardia of 230 per minute, where the P waves are difficult to recognize with certainty, but now with S-T depressions. Thus, this is not an actual positive electrocardiographic exercise test but a supraventricular paroxysmal tachycardia, which in this patient appeared in particular after effort.

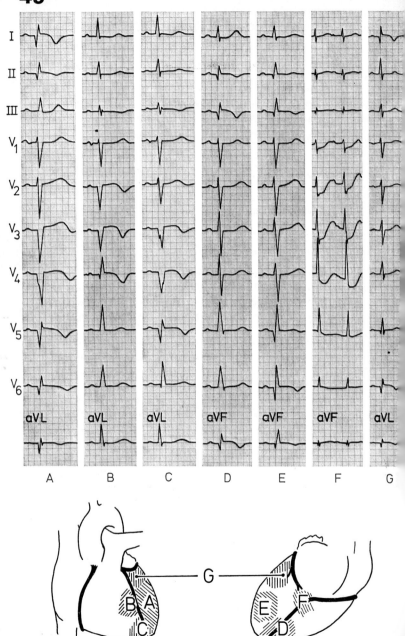

49*

ACUTE MYOCARDIAL INFARCTION 1

The development of the typical infarction pattern in leads facing a *transmural* infarction is as follows:

Commences with elevation of the S-T segment ("injury pattern").

Simultaneously, or a little later, a Q wave develops.

Gradually the elevation of S-T decreases, and at the same time, the T wave becomes first diphasic

and later negative, often with "coronary" shape.

The R wave may disappear completely, so that the QRS complex consists of only one so-called QS deflection.

In a *nontransmural* (subendocardial) infarction:

only changes in the S-T segment and in the T waves are seen. Such infarcts can be diagnosed only by series electrocardiography and comparison with clinical findings.

49 Infarction localization is shown here schematically.

Anterior wall infarction. Infarction patterns in the precordial leads and often in I, II and aVL. **(A) Anterolateral.** Large infarction, seen in V_{3-6}, I(-II) and aVL. **(B) Anteroseptal.** More limited, seen in V_{2-3}, possibly also slightly in V_1 and V_4. **(C) Anteroapical.** More limited, seen in V_{3-5}. There can also be infarction patterns in I and aVL.

Posterior wall infarction. Infarction pattern in III, II and aVF and certain changes in precordial leads. **(D) Inferior** (syn. posteroinferior, diaphragmatic), seen in III, II and aVF. **(E) Inferolateral** (syn. posterolateral), seen in III, II, aVF and V_6, possibly also in V_5. **(F) Posterior** (syn. true posterior, posteroseptal, posterobasal). Often difficult to diagnose. Known in practice as "inverted infarction pattern" in precordial leads: S-T depressions and *relatively* (in relation to the normal, especially the patient's own previous recordings) tall, possibly wide R waves (typical infarction patterns may be elicited in leads from the back).

Lateral infarction (G) (syn. laterobasal), seen in V_6, I and aVL.

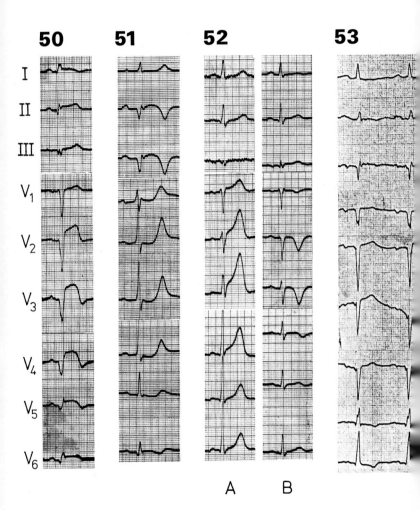

ACUTE MYOCARDIAL INFARCTION 2

Various localizations of the infarction (see p. 67) can naturally appear combined. Multiple infarcts can show combined patterns, or these may partly cancel each other, so that the changes may be modest in relation to the size of the infarction, possibly with low voltage.

In addition to localization and depth (transmural/nontransmural), infarction can be characterized by the stage and by complicating dysrhythmias. Atrioventricular block is seen particularly in posterior wall infarction (atrioventricular node arterial supply), sinoatrial block and other bradyarrhythmias likewise especially in posterior wall infarction. possibly also in lateral infarction (the sinoatrial node arterial supply). Tachyarrhythmias are seen in all types. Bundle branch block is seen in particular in infarction that involves the septum (see p. 71).

50 **Anterolateral infarction** in early stage. Typical changes in I, II and $V_{(2-)3-6}$.

51 **Inferolateral infarction** in slightly later stage. Changes in III, II and V_6. The stage is one of inverted T waves of "coronary"shape. The example shows, in addition, "mirror-image patterns" in other leads (V_{1-5}).

52 **Subendocardial infarction** (anteroseptal). (A) First day. (B) Twentieth day. The changes appear only in the S-T segments and T waves. However, decreasing amplitude of the R waves is seen, but no Q waves.

53 **Multiple infarcts.** Q waves are seen in III and QS waves in V_{1-4} but very small changes in the S-T segment and T waves. Resembles anteroseptal and inferior changes of older date. Autopsy showed a large, fresh inferior infarction and anterior and posterior infarcts about a month old. Almost no healthy myocardial tissue left.

54

55*

56*

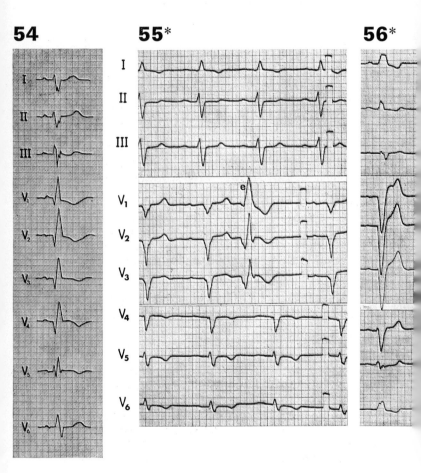

ACUTE MYOCARDIAL INFARCTION
AND BUNDLE BRANCH BLOCK

Infarction of the septum can give rise to acute bundle branch block.

In preexisting left bundle branch block, the electrocardiographic diagnosis of myocardial infarction is difficult or impossible. The reason is that left bundle branch block (and pronounced left ventricular hypertrophy) in itself can give rise to a QS-like pattern in V_{1-3} and III, as the R waves in these leads can be minimal or missing. In addition, when left bundle branch block is present, Q waves usually will be lacking in the "left leads" I and V_{5-6}, even in anterior infarction. Finally, the bundle branch block in itself results in pronounced S-T and T changes, which may mask the infarct changes. At times, extrasystoles from the left ventricle can be of diagnostic help.

In preexisting right bundle branch block, on the other hand, a diagnosis of infarction often is rather easy, as an anterior infarction gives Q waves with increasing amplitude from V_1 in over the precordium, and an inferior infarction gives large and wide Q waves in II and III, which do not belong to the typical picture of right bundle branch block.

54 Scheme showing the **typical pattern of anterior infarction in right bundle branch block.** Characteristic are large Q waves, increasing in amplitude from V_1 in over the precordium. As a result of the bundle branch block, the same leads maintain tall and wide R waves.

55 60-year-old man with **left bundle branch block.** History suggested coronary occlusion 1 year before, and there are QS waves in V_{1-3} and a minimal R wave in V_4; but as left bundle branch block in itself can give a similar pattern, the diagnosis is uncertain. The extrasystole e, which has a configuration like right bundle branch block and thus originates from the left ventricle, shows, however, that this is an **old anterior infarction,** as e has large Q waves that increase from V_1 to V_3.

56 **Left bundle branch block** in patient **without myocardial infarction.** The figure is included in order to show the great similarity between QRS in V_{1-3} in this case and in **55.** There is a large QS wave in V_{1-2} but admittedly a minimal initial R wave in V_3.

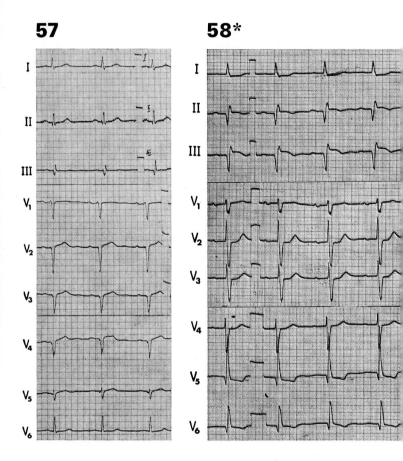

57

I

II

III

V₁

V₂

V₃

V₄

V₅

V₆

58*

I

II

III

V₁

V₂

V₃

V₄

V₅

V₆

PREVIOUS MYOCARDIAL INFARCTION

Among the typical changes in acute myocardial infarction (see p. 67), the *S-T displacements* are the most transient, and as a rule they disappear in the course of days to a fortnight.

During the weeks or months after the acute infarction, the coronary *T waves* usually will show a tendency to become flatter, and finally they can return to normal.

Coronary *Q waves* (or QS waves) are the most permanent features and often will be found for years in leads over scars after myocardial infarction.

The electrocardiographic picture of an *old healed infarction,* therefore, will be characterized by Q waves over the affected region, often with flattened or slightly negative T waves.

If S-T elevations together with Q waves persist unchanged for months to years following an acute infarction, one may suspect *aneurysm of the ventricular wall.*

57   **Old infarction.** Electrocardiogram from a patient who 2 years previously had a large anterior infarction. QS waves persist in leads V_{2-4} and qrS pattern in V_5, but all the changes in the S-T segments and T waves have disappeared.

58   **Ventricular aneurysm** below on the back wall of the left ventricle following an inferior infarction. The patient was a 71-year-old man who 3 years previously had been admitted to the hospital for acute coronary occlusion.

The electrocardiogram shows large Q waves in II and III but at the same time considerable S-T elevation with slight inversion of T in the same leads – and corresponding S-T depression in I and V_{2-5}. Review of the old case records showed that these S-T displacements had remained unchanged during the course of the 3 years, and an x-ray examination with kymography confirmed the diagnosis of left ventricular aneurysm.

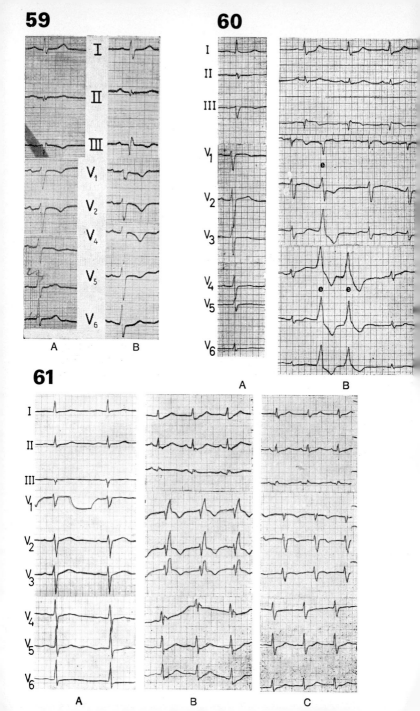

59

A   B

I
II
III
V₁
V₂
V₄
V₅
V₆

60

I
II
III
V₁
V₂
V₃
V₄
V₅
V₆

A   B

61

I
II
III
V₁
V₂
V₃
V₄
V₅
V₆

A   B   C

PULMONARY EMBOLISM

The characteristic electrocardiographic features are:

(1) *Shift of the electrical axis to the right.* This need not result in right axis deviation; the axis often merely turns slightly as a result of dilatation of the right ventricle, seen as an increase in size of the S wave in lead I. In addition, a large Q wave often is seen in lead III.

(2) *Acute right heart dilatation.* In severe cases, this is revealed by an acute occurrence of incomplete or complete right bundle branch block (see pp. 53 and 51). In milder cases there merely is seen increasing amplitude of the S wave in V_{5-6}.

(3) *Inversion of T waves in III and V_{1-3}.* In addition, displacements of S-T can be seen in the form of elevation in III and depression in I, II and V_{1-3}.

(4) *Acute occurrence of arrhythmias* such as extrasystoles, atrial fibrillation or atrial flutter.

The electrocardiogram in pulmonary embolism can resemble that of inferior myocardial infarction, especially if in lead III there is a large Q wave, elevation of S-T and inversion of the T wave. However, pulmonary embolism usually is distinguished by the following: (1) The changes are more transient. (2) Increasing S wave in I and V_6. (3) No Q wave in lead II.

59 **Pulmonary embolism.** (A) The electrocardiogram is seen before the attack. (B) Just after the acute attack, a shift of the axis to the right is seen (increasing S_I and R_{III}), large Q_{III} and increasing inversion of the T wave in $V_{1-2-4-5}$ (V_3 omitted) and increasing amplitude of the S wave in V_{5-6}.

60 **Pulmonary embolism.** Electrocardiogram before the attack (A) shows left axis deviation. Immediately after the acute attack (B), axis shift to the right is seen (S_I), large Q_{III}, depressed S-T in I and V_3 (and suggested in II), elevation of S-T_{III} and ventricular extrasystoles (e).

61 **Pulmonary embolism.** (A) A normal electrocardiogram is seen before the acute attack. Curve (B) was taken ½ hour after an acute severe attack, which clinically resembled pulmonary embolism. Right bundle branch block is seen and small Q_{III}. Three hours later (C), the bundle branch block had disappeared, but large S waves persist in I and V_{5-6} and the T inversion in V_{1-3}. (Artifact in V_1 of curve A.)

75

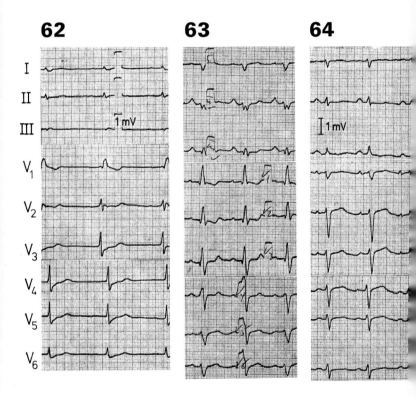

CHRONIC COR PULMONALE

The electrocardiogram does not provide a constant diagnostic means for the right ventricular hypertrophy in chronic pulmonary disease with cor pulmonale.

Enlargement of the right atrium is manifested by "P pulmonale" (see p. 45).

Electrocardiographic signs of *affection of the right ventricle* are most typically present in the form of right bundle branch block (complete or incomplete) or signs of hypertrophy of the right ventricle.

A number of patients show only a pronounced *"emphysema electrocardiogram"* with P pulmonale, right axis deviation, S waves right out to the lateral precordial leads and low voltage of QRS.

In the type of chronic cor pulmonale that is due to *primary* lung vessel disease, clear signs of hypertrophy of the right ventricle are more frequent.

62 Chronic cor pulmonale with right bundle branch block.
Man aged 71 years with chronic bronchitis, pulmonary emphysema and pulmonary cancer has pulmonary hypertension (systolic 40-50 mm Hg) at rest and peripheral edema. The electrocardiogram shows right bundle branch block at the boundary between complete and incomplete (QRS = 0.10-0.12 second; cf. pp. 51-53) and low voltage in I-III.

63 Chronic cor pulmonale with pronounced right ventricular hypertrophy.
Man aged 41 years with obstructive lung disease for 20 years and severe manifest right congestive heart failure. Pronounced right axis deviation and right ventricular hypertrophy are seen (tall R in V_1), P pulmonale, large S wave in V_{3-6}, low voltage in I-III and sinus tachycardia.

64 Chronic cor pulmonale with "emphysema electrocardiogram".
Woman aged 65 years with chronic obstructive pulmonary disease, enlarged heart and moderate right congestive heart failure. Right axis deviation is seen. There is no clear-cut right ventricular hypertrophy, but large S waves in all precordial leads. The P waves are largest in II and III as in P pulmonale, but without exceeding the boundaries for normal. Low voltage and sinus tachycardia. Also compare **21**, page 45.

65

I

II

III

V₁

V₂

V₃

V₄

V₅

V₆

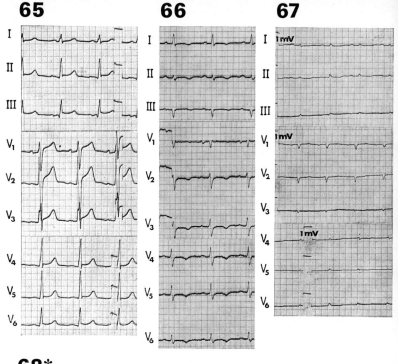

66

I

II

III

V₁

V₂

V₃

V₄

V₅

V₆

67

I · 1 mV

II

III

V₁ · 1 mV

V₂

V₃

V₄ · 1 mV

V₅

V₆

68*

I · 1 mV

II

III

V₁

V₂

V₃

V₄

V₅

V₆

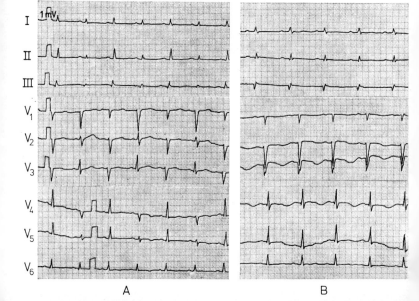

A

B

ACUTE PERICARDITIS

In pericarditis, changes usually are seen in the standard limb leads and in those precordial leads that face the affected part of the pericardium. As pericarditis frequently is diffuse, changes often are seen in all leads. The changes are:

(1) *Elevation of S-T segment.* Usually after a few days, the elevation regresses and, in most cases, the following changes then develop.
(2) *Inversion of T wave.* In some cases, only T inversion is seen without preceding S-T elevation.
(3) In pericardial effusion, *low voltage of QRS complex and T wave* often are seen.

In pericarditis, no Q waves or QS waves are seen as is the case in acute myocardial infarction. The changes, however, resemble those in nontransmural infarction (see p. 67), so that series electrocardiography is important. In pericarditis, the development of the electrocardiographic changes usually takes place more slowly than in myocardial infarction.

65 Acute diffuse dry pericarditis. Elevation of the S-T segment is seen in all leads, least pronounced in I.

66 Acute diffuse dry pericarditis in a later stage. Inversion of the T wave in all leads except V_1.

67 Subacute diffuse exudative pericarditis with massive pericardial effusion. There is pronounced low voltage of all waves in all leads (note the correct mV test). In addition, sinus tachycardia, rate about 125 per minute.

68 Pericardial effusion with electrical alternans. By electrical alternans is understood sinus rhythm with alternation in the amplitude of QRS. It now is also well known that electrical alternans can be a characteristic finding in pericardial effusion, particularly in the malignant form. The mechanism still is being discussed. (A) Electrical alternans, so pronounced that QRS changes main direction from beat to beat. In addition, flat T waves are seen and a tendency to low voltage. (B) After removal of 1900 ml pericardial fluid, the alternans phenomenon has disappeared, but low voltage and S-T changes persist.

69

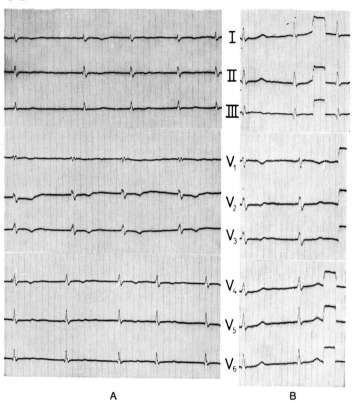

A

B

CHRONIC CONSTRICTIVE PERICARDITIS
(CONSTRICTIO CORDIS)

The thickened shell of fibrous, possibly also calcified, pericardium produces the characteristic (1) *low voltage of QRS* in all leads. In addition there are changes in the T waves that resemble those in acute pericarditis: (2) *Flat* or inverted *T waves.* Frequently there are in addition (3) wide P waves or *atrial fibrillation.*

69 Younger woman with **chronic constrictive pericarditis.** (A) The electrocardiogram shows low voltage in all leads, atrial fibrillation with slow ventricular response and T changes in the form of flat to diphasic T waves in I, II, III V₁, V₅ and V₆ and T inversion in V₂₋₄. (B) The electrocardiogram from the same patient 1½ year after successful pericardiectomy. The amplitude of the QRS complexes has increased and the T waves now are practically normal. There still is atrial fibrillation.

70*

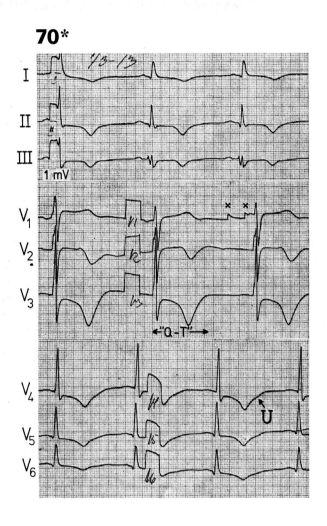

CEREBROVASCULAR ACCIDENT PATTERN

Following cerebrovascular accidents (subarachnoid hemorrhage, cerebral hemorrhage, cerebral thrombosis, etc.), a characteristic electrocardiographic pattern may be observed in several cases, comprising *deep inversion of the T waves and pronounced U waves,* which can coalesce with the T waves. Often, a prolonged Q-T interval can be measured, although in reality this may be a long Q-U interval. At the same time there often is bradycardia.

In pronounced cases, an acute myocardial infarction is an obvious differential diagnosis. In cerebrovascular cases, major changes often appear early, and these persist strikingly unchanged for several days.

Myocardial damage has been demonstrated experimentally in intracranial hemorrhage. However, the mechanism in the development of these electrocardiographic changes is uncertain.

70 **Cerebrovascular accident pattern.** Electrocardiogram from a 59-year-old man 24 hours after the development of acute hemiplegia as a sequel to thrombosis of the right middle cerebral artery. Large T inversion in all leads with the exception of V_1, and at the same time S-T depression in several leads. The T waves coalesce with the U waves, so that the Q-T interval (= Q-U) is lengthened, calculated in V_3 as Q-T_c = 0.59 second (> 0.425; see p. 22). There are Q waves in several leads, but they are small, not "coronary", and serum enzymes did not suggest myocardial infarction. There is sinus bradycardia in V_{1-3}. (Artifact, marked x, in V_1.)

71

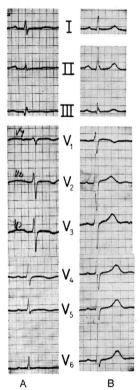

I

II

III

V$_1$

V$_2$

V$_3$

V$_4$

V$_5$

V$_6$

A   B

Myxedema often is accompanied by electrocardiographic changes, which can include (1) *bradycardia,* (2) lengthening of the P-R interval, (3) *low voltage of the QRS* complex and (4) *flat T waves.*

71   **Myxedema.** (A) Electrocardiogram from a 55-year-old woman with myxedema, basal metabolic rate 78% of normal. Low voltage of the QRS complexes and flat – in several leads inverted – T waves are seen. The P-R interval is not lengthened = 0.19 second. (B) Electrocardiogram from the same patient during adequate compensatory treatment. The amplitude of the QRS complex has increased in all leads, and the T waves now are normal. P-R interval is shorter, now 0.16 second.

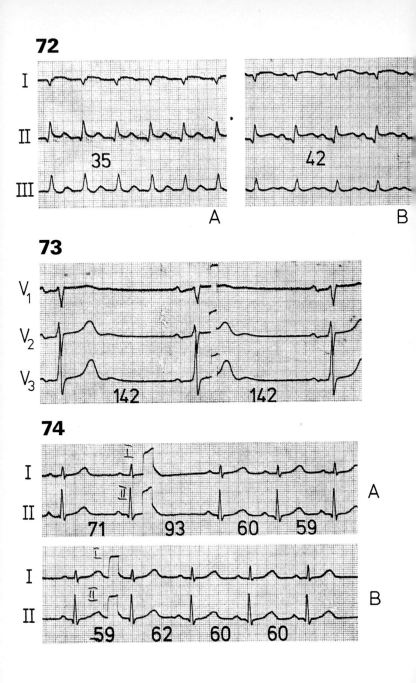

Normally, the sinoatrial node is the pacemaker of the heart, with a rate of 60-100 per minute.

Sinus rhythm with a rate above resp. below this range is by definition sinus tachycardia resp. sinus bradycardia.

Sinus rhythm rarely is completely regular. The designation sinus arrhythmia is used commonly when the irregularity reaches a certain degree; e.g., if the difference between the largest and smallest P-P intervals (and thereby the R-R interval) is at least 0.12 second or if the P-P intervals vary by 10% or more. Sinus arrhythmia most often is respiratory arrhythmia, which is most common in children and elderly people. More rarely, sinus arrhythmia is independent of respiration, most often with longer periods of relatively rapid or slow rate.

The most important feature of sinus arrhythmia is to remember that it occurs normally, also in other disturbances of rhythm. It therefore is not necessary to demand completely regular rhythm as a sign of sinoatrial node activity in the interpretation of dysrhythmias; see, for example, **110,** page 102.

72 **Sinus tachycardia.** (A) The R-R interval is 35 hundredths of a second, so that the rate is about 170/min. Patient with severe heart failure during acute anterior infarction. The P waves are not clearly seen so that on this recording alone it cannot be seen whether this is a case of sinus tachycardia. (B) The rate decreased slowly during treatment, and it now is seen that the P waves in recording A must have been hidden within the T waves. Now, sinus tachycardia with a rate of 143/min.

73 **Sinus bradycardia.** The R-R intervals are 142 hundredths of a second, so that the frequency is 42/min.

74 **Sinus arrhythmia.** (A) The R-R intervals are given in hundredths of a second. The difference between the longest and the shortest interval is 0.34 second. Child with respiratory arrhythmia. (B) The patient is holding his breath, and the sinus rhythm is more regular.

75

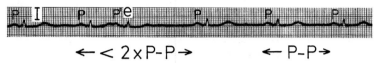

$\leftarrow < 2 \times P\text{-}P \rightarrow$ $\leftarrow P\text{-}P \rightarrow$

76

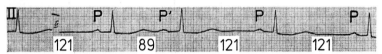

77

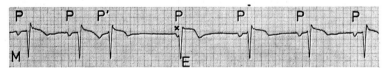

78

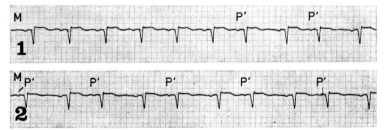

79*

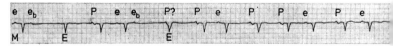

80

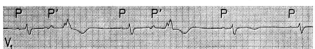

ATRIAL EXTRASYSTOLES

Atrial extrasystoles are heartbeats that arise in an ectopic atrial focus abnormally early in the basic rhythm ("premature beats"). They present in the form of a premature P wave of deviant form. If the impulse is transmitted to the ventricles, the P-R interval is more than 0.12 second. The interval after the extrasystole often is longer than the P-P interval in basic rhythm but frequently not fully compensatory (cf. p. 24).

75 **Atrial extrasystole.** In the extrasystole (e), the P wave (P′) is of a shape other than in the sinus beats (P), P′-R $>$ 0.12 second, and QRS is of normal shape. The compensatory pause is incomplete; i.e., the distance between the preceding and following beats is $<$ 2 $\times$ P-P.

76 **Atrial extrasystole without compensatory pause.** The third beat is an atrial extrasystole: it arrives too early and has a slightly widened P wave (P′). The post-extrasystolic interval is equal to the following interval (R-R intervals in hundredths of a second).

77 **Atrial extrasystole with long compensatory pause and junctional escape beat.** The third beat is an atrial extrasystole (P′ too early and of deviant shape). The post-extrasystolic pause is compensatory and so long that a junctional escape beat (E) appears before the P wave, marked x, manages to be transmitted.

78 **Multiple atrial extrasystoles.** Continuous strips 1 and 2. The atrial extrasystoles are shown with P′ waves. They result in bigeminy; i.e., every second beat is an extrasystole. Full compensatory pause.

79 **Blocked atrial extrasystoles.** Multiple atrial extrasystoles, marked e. Two of them, marked e_b, arrive so early that the atrioventricular node is refractory. Therefore, they are not transmitted to the ventricles and consist only of a P′ wave, and therefore are called blocked or nonconducted atrial extrasystoles. The beats E are escape beats; cf.**77**. The P waves of the sinus beats are marked P.

80 **Atrial extrasystoles with aberrant ventricular conduction.** Beats nos. 2 and 4 are atrial extrasystoles, as they are characterized by premature and abnormal P waves (P′). However, the impulse is transmitted to the ventricles in an abnormal manner: right bundle branch block pattern. Such atrial extrasystoles with aberrant conduction can be misinterpreted as ventricular extrasystoles, especially if P′ lies hidden within the preceding T wave.

81

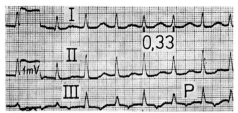

82

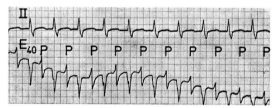

83

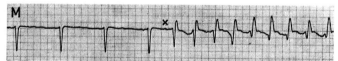

84*

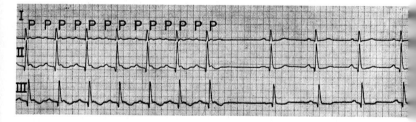

85

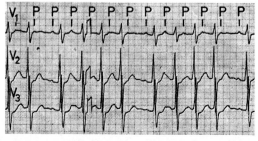

ATRIAL PAROXYSMAL TACHYCARDIA

Atrial paroxysmal tachycardia is the occurrence in attacks of a rapid, regular ectopic rhythm, usually with a rate in the range 160-250/min (in infants, an even more rapid rate can be seen). It is characterized by P waves of abnormal shape > 0.12 second preceding QRS. The rapid types are distinguished from atrial flutter by not having the typical saw-tooth baseline. The QRS complexes most often are of supraventricular (narrow) type.

81   **Atrial paroxysmal tachycardia.** Beginning with beat no. 2, tachycardia is seen with a rate of 180/min. Deformed P waves are clearly seen with P-R > 0.12 second.

82   **Atrial paroxysmal tachycardia.** Supraventricular tachycardia with a rate of 155/min is seen in II, but the P waves are not seen clearly. In the esophageal lead (E_{40}), the P waves appear with P-R > 0.12 second.

83   **Atrial paroxysmal tachycardia with aberrant ventricular conduction.** After four sinus beats, a tachycardia commences with a rate of 200-215/min. The QRS complexes have the shape of bundle branch block and therefore resemble ventricular tachycardia, but the tachycardia *begins* with a P wave (marked x), and the bundle branch block is of right-sided type. Therefore, this is a case of an atrial tachycardia, but with aberrant conduction to the ventricles (cf. **11**, p. 39).

84   **Atrial tachycardia with 2:1 atrioventricular block.** On closer examination, the tachycardia to the left, in addition to the distinct P waves, shows extra P waves just after QRS. The P rhythm is regular = 255/min. A rhythm of this kind can be erroneously diagnosed as sinus tachycardia. In cases of doubt, an esophageal lead will reveal the P waves and thereby the rhythm. Transition to sinus rhythm.

85   **Atrial tachycardia with atrioventricular block of Wenckebach type.** An atrial tachycardia is seen with a rate of 200/min. Wenckebach periods are seen (cf. **146**, p. 125), resulting in 5:4 atrioventicular block. The ventricular rhythm hereby becomes irregular. The differential diagnosis with respect to atrial fibrillation with rapid ventricular response is important, as atrial tachycardia with block often is due to digitalis.

86

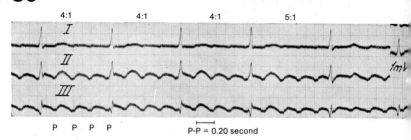

4:1   4:1   4:1   5:1

I

II

1mv

III

P   P   P   P

P-P = 0.20 second

87

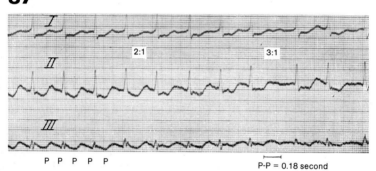

I

2:1   3:1

II

III

P   P   P   P   P

P-P = 0.18 second

88

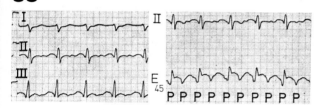

I   II

II

III   E₄₅

P P P P P P P P P P

89

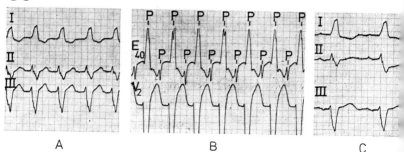

I   P P P P P P P   I

II   E₄₀   II

III   V₂   III

A   B   C

Atrial flutter is characterized by (1) a rapid, regular atrial rhythm, (2) atrial complexes of a "saw-toothed shape", especially in leads II and III, and (3) some degree of functional atrioventricular block (often regular). The saw-tooth baseline ("flutter waves", F waves) is explained as being a combination of negative ectopic P waves (P') and pronounced atrial repolarization waves (Ta); see sketch. The rate for flutter is commonly stated to vary from 250 to 400/min, most often 300 to 320. The distinction downward from atrial tachycardia and upward from atrial fibrillation, however, is not sharp.

86 **Atrial flutter with appropriate block.** The regular saw-toothed F waves (marked P) are seen most clearly in II and III. To the left, regular 4:1 block, giving a regular heart rhythm of 75/min on clinical examination. The flutter rate is 300/min.

87 **Atrial flutter with tachycardia.** To the left, 2:1 block, and both clinically and electrocardiographically, this condition is difficult to distinguish from atrial paroxysmal tachycardia. The varying block in the right-hand part of the curve shows that this is a case of atrial flutter. Atrial rate is 335/min.

88 **Atrial flutter with 2:1 block, resembling sinus tachycardia or supraventricular paroxysmal tachycardia.** Leads I-III show tachycardia of 130/min and the P waves are difficult to localize. An esophageal lead (E_{45}) shows atrial flutter of 270/min (marked P) and 2:1 block (patient with aortic valve disease and LPH; cf. p. 55).

89 **Atrial flutter with 2:1 block, differential diagnosis with respect to ventricular tachycardia.** (A) The standard limb leads show tachycardia 145/min with widened ventricular complexes, resembling ventricular tachycardia. (B) Esophageal lead (E_{40}) shows in several places P waves on the top of QRS (see in particular complexes nos. 2 and 4) exactly midway between the other P waves; in other words, atrial flutter with a rate of 300/min (the rate must have increased between A and B, as the ventricular rate now is 150/min). (C) During sinus rhythm, it is seen that this is a case of permanent left bundle branch block. (Differential diagnostic difficulties with respect to ventricular tachycardia may also arise if during atrial flutter there is aberrant ventricular conduction with bundle branch block pattern alone during the attack [cf. **83,** p. 90].)

90

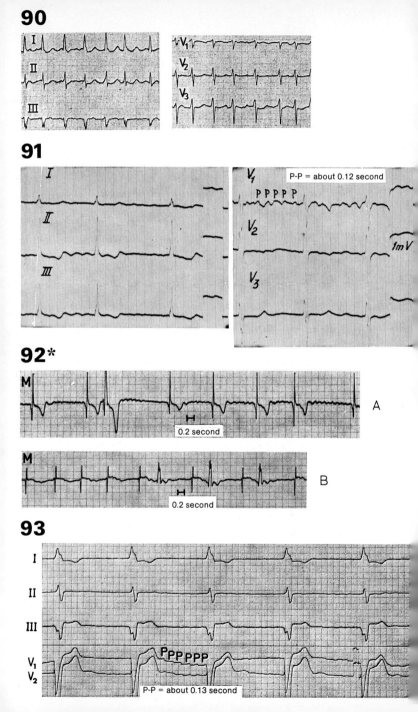

I II III V₁ V₂ V₃

91

I II III

V₁   P-P = about 0.12 second
P P P P P
V₂   1mV
V₃

92*

M   A
⊢ 0.2 second ⊣

M   B
⊢ 0.2 second ⊣

93

I II III

V₁ V₂   P P P P P P
P-P = about 0.13 second

ATRIAL FIBRILLATION

The atria can beat regularly with a rate of up to 350-400/min (see atrial flutter). If the rate increases further, the rhythm becomes irregular because of continuously varying ("chaotic") spread of the impulses. This condition is designated atrial fibrillation. It is seen on the electrocardiogram as an irregular baseline, which more or less clearly shows waves ("fibrillation waves", f waves). These can be seen best in leads that are near the atria (e.g., V_1). If it is possible from these to calculate a mean atrial rate, this will lie in the region (350)-400-700/min. The impulses reach the atrioventricular node with a high rate, but here there is a favorable functional block resulting in irregular ventricular response.

90 **Untreated atrial fibrillation with rapid ventricular response.** There is almost no visible atrial activity, not even in V_{1-3}. The ventricular rhythm is irregular, mean rate about 175/min.

91 **Atrial fibrillation with controlled ventricular rate in a digitalized patient.** The P waves occur irregularly (f waves, seen best in V_1). Mean atrial rate of about 500/min. Adequate slow ventricular arrhythmia.

92 **Atrial fibrillation with suspected aberrant conduction beats.** Aberrant ventricular conduction (see p. 23) is difficult to demonstrate with certainty in atrial fibrillation, but can be suspected if a ventricular beat (1) resembles right bundle branch block pattern and (2) terminates a short R-R interval, which follows after a long interval. (A) and (B) are from 2 patients with atrial fibrillation (wavy baseline). Beats no. 3 in (A) and nos. 6, 8 and 10 in (B) probably are aberrant conduction beats according to the criteria mentioned. In atrial fibrillation, however, it is never possible by means of conventional electrocardiography to be quite certain of the differential diagnosis with respect to ventricular extrasystoles.

93 **Atrial fibrillation simultaneously with third degree atrioventricular block.** This patient shows one of the rare cases of atrial fibrillation without ventricular arrhythmia. The fibrillation waves are clearly seen in V_1 (marked P), rate of about 460/min. Because of third degree atrioventricular block, the ventricles beat with a regular idioventricular rhythm, which arises in the right ventricle (resembles left bundle branch block), rate 46/min.

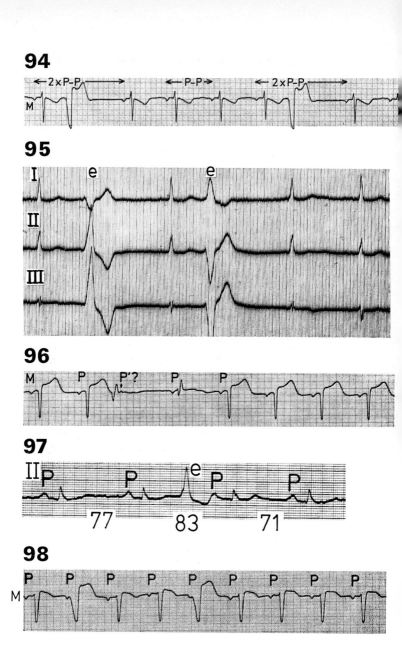

94

2 × P-P ← P-P → ← 2 × P-P

M

95

I   e   e

II

III

96

M   P   P'?   P   P

97

II P   P   e P   P

77   83   71

98

P P P P P P P P P

M

Ventricular extrasystoles usually are characterized by the following: They appear abnormally early in the rhythm ("premature beats"), QRS has a deviant shape and often a large amplitude, the T wave is directed opposite to the main deflection in QRS, there is complete compensatory pause and, finally, QRS usually is not related to a P wave. The shape of the QRS complex thus resembles the pattern in bundle branch block, and it often is possible from the shape to see from which ventricle the extrasystole comes: In extraxystoles from the right ventricle, QRS resembles left bundle branch block, and vice versa.

94 **Unifocal extrasystoles.** Beats nos. 2 and 7 appear too early, the shape is uniform and characteristic for ventricular beats. Complete compensatory pause; see P-P.

95 **Extrasystoles from both ventricles.** The first (2d beat) comes from a center in the left ventricle (QRS resembles that in right bundle branch block), the second (4th beat) from the right ventricle (resembles left bundle branch block).

96 **Post-extrasystolic aberrant conduction.** Beat no. 3 is a ventricular extrasystole. P'? indicates a presumed retrograde P wave from the extrasystole. The sinus beat following (no. 4) shows aberrant conduction to the ventricles, as it resembles right bundle branch block (cf. **11,** p. 39). This phenomenon most often is ascribed to transient "tiring" of the right bundle branch system after the retrograde conduction.

97 **Interpolated ventricular extrasystole.** The extrasystole (e) is "sandwiched" between two sinus beats. There is no compensatory pause, but the R-R interval in which the extrasystole is lying is slightly longer and the next interval is slightly shorter than the normal R-R interval (R-R intervals in hundredths of a second). This is due to a prolongation of the P-R interval following the extrasystole. The explanation is analogous with that under **96** (but here concealed conduction is assumed; see p. 25).

98 **End-diastolic ventricular extrasystoles.** Beats nos. 2 and 5 are ventricular extrasystoles; they appear too early, but only slightly so: they depolarize the ventricles just before the sinus impulse reaches the ventricles but after the sinus impulse has activated the atria.

99

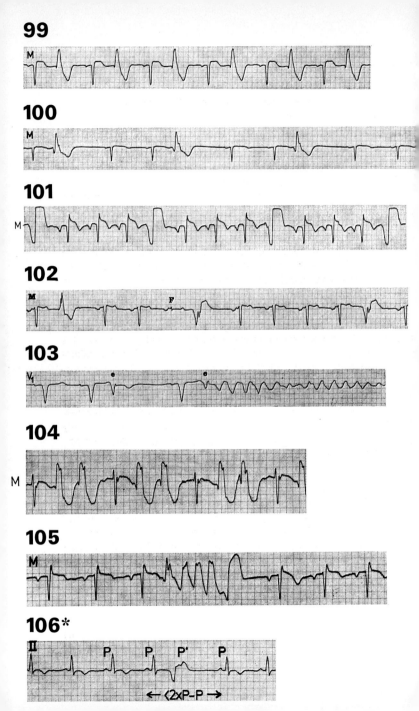

100

101

102

103

104

105

106*

VENTRICULAR EXTRASYSTOLES 2

99 Coupled ventricular extrasystoles with bigeminy. Each second beat is an extrasystole.

100 Coupled ventricular extrasystoles with trigeminy. Each third beat is a ventricular extrasystole.

101 Coupled ventricular extrasystoles with quadrigeminy. Each fourth beat is an extrasystole (S-T distorted).

102 Multifocal ventricular extrasystoles and fusion beats. By multifocal extrasystoles is understood extrasystoles from at least two foci. The complexes nos. 2, 6 and 11 are ventricular extrasystoles from two foci. Complex no. 5 (marked F) is a so-called fusion beat, which has originated by the ventricles being simultaneously activated from the sinoatrial node and from an extrasystolic center in the ventricles. QRS therefore becomes small and of short duration whereas the repolarization (T wave and Q-T interval) is normal. Note normal P-R interval in the fusion beat, in contrast to the beats in **98.**

103 Ventricular extrasystoles of "R on T type". Hereby is understood that the R wave of an extrasystole (or possibly the Q wave) is superimposed on the T wave of a preceding beat. Since the vulnerable period is, roughly speaking, around the top of a T wave, there is a risk that such an extrasystole will trigger off a ventricular tachycardia or ventricular fibrillation, especially in myocardial infarction. The beats (e) are of "R (here Q) on T type"; no. 2 starts ventricular fibrillation.

104 Ventricular extrasystoles in pairs. Here, extrasystoles occur in pairs, involving trigemini (of a morphology other than in **100**); involves a risk of ventricular fibrillation in acute myocardial infarction, as no. 2 in a pair easily becomes of the R on T type in relation to no. 1.

105 Run of ventricular extrasystoles. After the 3d beat there is a run of 5 extrasystoles; has the same ominous significance as **104.**

106 Ventricular extrasystole with retrograde conduction to the atria. Beat no. 5 is a ventricular extrasystole, which is conducted retrogradely to the atria (P') and "resets" the sinoatrial node: the distance from P' to the following P wave = the basic P-P interval; therefore, no complete compensatory pause. Retrograde conduction is the exception in ventricular extrasystoles.

107*

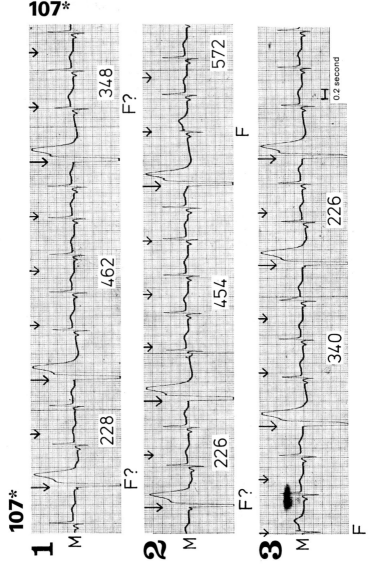

100

Parasystole is a disturbance of rhythm characterized by two centers constantly competing for control of the heart. One of the centers is the sinoatrial node; the other is an ectopic center, which is able to function at its own regular rhythm because in one way or another (called "entrance block") it is protected against being discharged (depolarized) by the sinoatrial node impulses. Conversely, the sinoatrial node continues to function undisturbed. Depending on the localization of the ectopic center, one speaks of atrial, junctional and ventricular parasystole. The last type is the most common.

The presence of ventricular parasystole is suspected when (1) "ventricular extrasystoles" from the same focus appear with strongly varying distance from the preceding sinus beat ("coupling interval") and (2) fusion beats are seen. Certainty is obtained if (3) a constant inherent rate can be calculated, fitting in with both the "ventricular extrasystoles" and the fusion beats. Ventricular parasystole is common in (caused by) fixed-rate artificial pacemaker treatment during periods without atrioventricular block; see, for example, **162,** page 131.

107

107 **Ventricular parasystole.** A series of beats is seen with characteristics as ventricular extrasystoles. Measuring (intervals are indicated in hundredths of a second) shows that these beats arise with a mutual distance that is a multiple of an interval of 1.13-1.16 seconds ($228 = 114 \times 2$; $462 = 116 \times 4$; $348 = 116 \times 3$; etc.). The basic rhythm for the parasystolic center that can be derived from these figures is marked by arrows. Only when these impulses are discharged outside the refractory period of the ventricles after the sinus beats can they depolarize the ventricles and give the characteristic "ventricular" beats (longer arrows). Occasionally the ventricles are depolarized simultaneously from the sinoatrial node and from the parasystolic focus, resulting in fusion beats. Two obvious fusion beats are marked with F, probable fusion beats with F?.

Continuous strips 1-3.

108

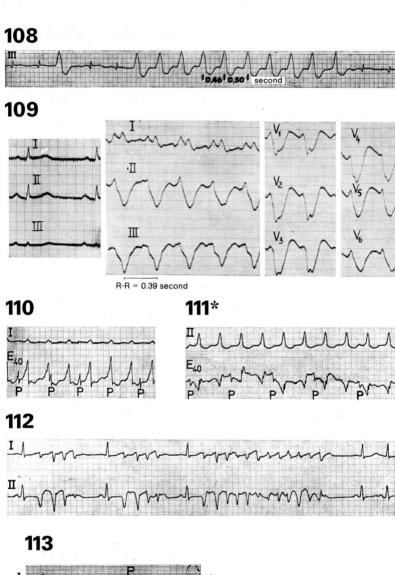

109

R-R = 0.39 second

110

111*

112

113

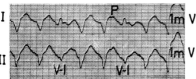

VENTRICULAR TACHYCARDIA

In ventricular tachycardia, the QRS complexes are of "ventricular" form, "wide and bizarre." The rate most often is 140-180/min, but 100-220 or more is seen; cf., however, ventricular flutter. The rhythm can be *slightly* irregular, the QRS configuration *slightly* varying. The P waves usually are impossible to see without an esophageal lead, which in most cases will show atrioventricular dissociation, but retrograde conduction to the atria may occur.

The differential diagnosis with regard to supraventricular tachycardia in a patient with bundle branch block or aberrant ventricular conduction often is difficult. Features in favor of ventricular tachycardia are: Start of an attack with a ventricular extrasystole, QRS shape (cf. **83,** p. 91), ventricular capture beats, fusion beats, atrioventricular dissociation.

108 **Ventricular tachycardia of brief duration.** Following a ventricular extrasystole, a short run of tachycardia (10 beats) is seen from the same focus, slight irregular rhythm, rate 120-130/min.

109 **Ventricular tachycardia in acute anterior infarction.** The infarction gives slight S-T elevation in I and II (the curve to the left). During the attack, wide, bizarre QRS complexes, rate 155/min. P waves cannot be distinguished.

110 **Ventricular tachycardia.** Esophageal lead (E_{40}) shows atrioventricular dissociation; in other words, the tachycardia is ventricular.

111 **Ventricular tachycardia.** Esophageal lead (E_{40}) shows a P wave for each second QRS complex, presumably due to retrograde conduction to the atria with 2:1 block.

112 **Repetitive ventricular tachycardia.** The distinction between runs of ventricular extrasystoles and brief ventricular tachycardia can be a question of definition. Here are two runs of 4 ventricular extrasystoles and then a run of 12 beats. This "multifocal" type of repetitive ventricular tachycardia sometimes is named "torsade de pointe."

113 **Ventricular tachycardia with ventricular capture beats.** The rhythm is interrupted several times by conducted sinus beats, which "capture" the ventricles. The ventricular capture beats, here marked V-I, have a deviant configuration and appear slightly early, and in one place the corresponding P wave is seen.

114

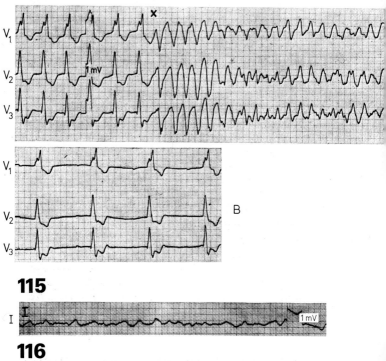

B

115

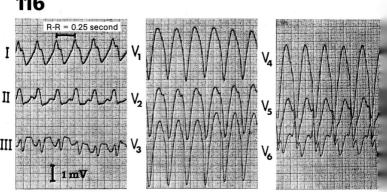

I   1 mV

116

R-R = 0.25 second

I   V₁   V₄

II   V₂   V₅

III V₃   V₆

1 mV

VENTRICULAR FIBRILLATION AND VENTRICULAR FLUTTER

Ventricular fibrillation is a state where the ventricles show quite weak, uncoordinated contractions whose pumping effect is zero. The electrocardiogram shows oscillations of continually varying amplitude and rate, most often in the range 200-600/min. At times, a distinction is made between fibrillation with large ("coarse fibrillation") and with small oscillations ("fine fibrillation").

By *ventricular flutter* is understood a state with more or less regular ventricular rhythm of 200-300/min where in most or all leads the electrocardiogram shows only diphasic deflections, in which it is difficult or impossible to recognize QRS. In reality, it is a very rapid ventricular tachycardia (cf. p. 103) with some pumping effect. It is reversible, but has a considerable tendency to pass into ventricular fibrillation.

114 **Ventricular fibrillation.** (A) At the right, tachycardia is seen with wide complexes, resembling ventricular tachycardia. At ✕, it converts to ventricular flutter and immediately to (coarse) ventricular fibrillation. (B) After electrical defibrillation, sinus rhythm is seen with a long P-R interval. QRS shows right bundle branch block of the same type as at the beginning of curve A. The tachycardia to the left in curve A thus has been supraventricular.

115 **Ventricular fibrillation** with small oscillations: "fine" fibrillation.

116 **Ventricular flutter.** In V_{1-6}, large, diphasic deflections are seen without recognizable QRS complexes, rate 240/min.

117

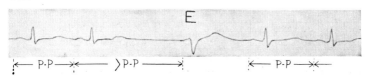

118

119

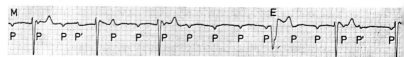

120

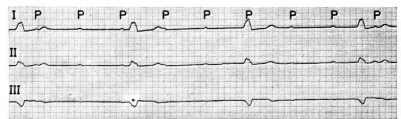

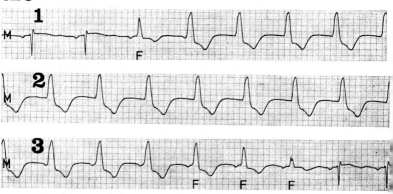

121

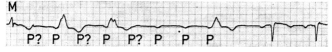

VENTRICULAR ESCAPE RHYTHMS

These comprise ventricular escape beats and idioventricular rhythms. The escape beat occurs after a pause in the basic rhythm (that is, late in contrast to the extrasystole) and "saves the heart from standstill." As a rule, idioventricular rhythm has a slow rate, but in coronary monitoring, it has been found in recent years that especially in acute myocardial infarction a more rapid idioventricular rhythm of 50-100/min can appear. It is called here accelerated idioventricular rhythm (syn.: idioventricular tachycardia).

117 **Ventricular escape beat.** After two sinus beats, sinoatrial block occurs, and after a pause (escape interval > P-P) there is an escape beat E, with "ventricular" shape.

118 **Ventricular escape beat.** Atrioventricular third degree block. The ventricles are driven by a junctional center, but after the first three beats there is a standstill in this rhythm and, after a pause, the ventricular escape beat E appears. (The P waves are missing in two places, presumably because of atrial extrasystoles, marked P'.)

119 **Idioventricular rhythm.** Third degree atrioventricular block. The ventricles are controlled by an idioventricular escape rhythm with the usual slow rate (about 32/min), presumably from the right ventricle (resembles left bundle branch block).

120 **Accelerated idioventricular rhythm.** In this patient with acute myocardial infarction there is a ventricular center with its own inherent rate of about 72/min, which has an opportunity to appear when the sinus rate is retarded and is once again depressed by the sinus rhythm when the rate of this increases. There is atrioventricular dissociation during the idioventricular rhythm because of retrograde block from the ventricles to the atria. Continuous strips 1-3: At the beginning, two sinus beats. The P-P interval increases, and the third beat is a fusion beat (F); the ventricles are depolarized simultaneously from the sinus node and the ventricular center. After this, the accelerated idioventricular rhythm is seen up to the middle of the curve strip 3, where the sinoatrial node speeds up; after three fusion beats (F), once more there is sinus rhythm.

121 **Irregular idioventricular rhythm.** Atrial or sinus tachycardia with third degree atrioventricular block. The ventricles are maintained in action by ventricular escape beats from various centers. To the right, conducted beats.

122

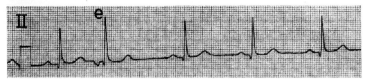

123

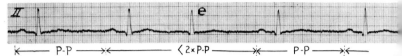

124*

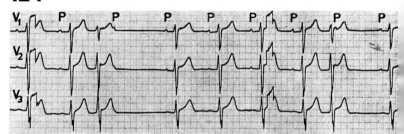

125

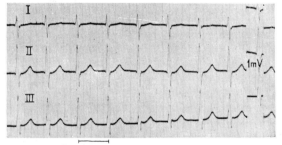

R-R = 0.45 second

126

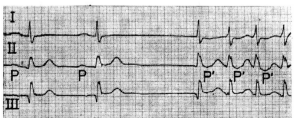

JUNCTIONAL EXTRASYSTOLES
AND TACHYCARDIA

Improved knowledge of the structure and function of the atrioventricular transition zone of the conduction system has resulted in terminologic diversities. Instead of the old terms nodal or atrioventricular nodal or AV nodal for ectopic rhythms from this area many prefer the broad designation atrioventricular junctional or junctional. In this atlas, the term junctional is used. The old terms upper, middle and lower (nodal resp. junctional) are abandoned, as not only the site of the ectopic center but also the rate of spread of the impulse in both directions determines the position of P in relation to QRS.

Junctional beats are characterized by QRS resembling the QRS of the sinus rhythm and by P of retrograde shape, i.e., negative in the leads, where sinus rhythm P waves are positive, and vice versa. P precedes QRS with P-R < 0.12 second or P is hidden in QRS or P lies just after QRS.

122 Junctional extrasystole. QRS in the extrasystole (e) resembles the QRS of the sinus beats, P is retrograde and P-R < 0.12 second.

123 Junctional extrasystole. QRS in the extrasystole (e) resembles QRS of the sinus beats. P is not seen. Incomplete compensatory pause (as in **122**).

124 Junctional extrasystoles with retrograde block ("main stem extrasystoles"). Beats nos. 3 and 8 are extrasystoles of supraventricular configuration. There must be retrograde block to the atria, as the P waves of the sinus rhythm continue unchanged. It has been the opinion that the focus is in the main stem of the bundle of His.

125 Junctional paroxysmal tachycardia. The QRS complexes are of the same type as in the patient's normal electrocardiogram. P waves not seen. Rate 135/min. It is difficult without special leads (e.g., esophageal) to maintain that this is not a case of an atrial tachycardia with P hidden within T and long P-R.

126 Junctional paroxysmal tachycardia. If, as here, we have the start of a paroxysmal supraventricular tachycardia, it often is possible to decide whether it is atrial or junctional. The first two beats show sinus rhythm with lengthened P-R. After a pause, a tachycardia commences with QRS of supraventricular type. It is junctional, as the first beat is not preceded by a P wave. Retrograde P waves (P') can just be noticed after QRS. The last three beats show slight aberration.

127*

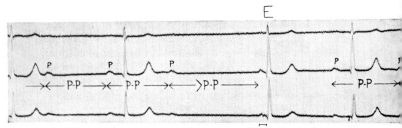

E

P   P   P   P   P

←— P-P —→←— P-P —→←—— P-P ——→   ←— P-P —→

P-R = 0.11 second

128

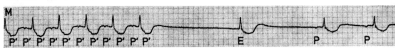

M

P' P' P' P' P' P' P' P' P' P'   E   P   P

129

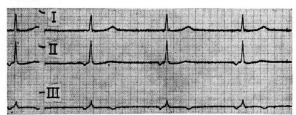

I

II

III

130

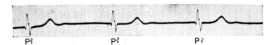

P?   P?   P?

131

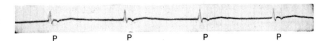

P   P̄   P   P

132*

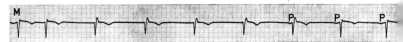

M   P   P   P

JUNCTIONAL ESCAPE RHYTHMS

These, in analogy with ventricular escape rhythms (see p. 107), comprise *junctional escape beats and junctional rhythm.* The inherent rate of the junctional rhythm most often is 40-60/min. However, more rapid rhythms are known in the range between these rates and those that are characteristic of paroxysmal tachycardia. Such rhythms are called "nonparoxysmal junctional tachycardia" or "*accelerated* idiojunctional rhythm." An example of this is seen in **163,** page 133.

127 **Junctional escape beat.** The patient has second degree atrioventricular block. In the middle of the curve, sinus arrest occurs and, after a pause (escape interval $>$ P-P), escape beat E appears, after which the sinoatrial node takes up its activity again (once more P waves). The fact that the escape is junctional is seen from QRS showing only slight aberration, P being small and deformed and P-R $<$ 0.12 second (leads I-III).

128 **Junctional escape beat.** To the left, atrial tachycardia, rate 220/min with 2:1 atrioventricular block. When it stops, sinoatrial block or sinus arrest develops, but the heart is "saved from standstill" by the junctional escape beat E, and after a further pause the sinoatrial node takes up its function again (the last two beats). Cf. also **157,** page 127

129 **Junctional rhythm.** P waves of retrograde type (negative in II and III) and P-R $<$ 0.12 second. Rate 57/min.

130 **Junctional rhythm.** P waves not seen, presumably hidden within QRS (lead II).

131 **Junctional rhythm.** Deformed ("retrograde") P waves after QRS (lead II).

132 **Periodic junctional rhythm with retrograde block (idiojunctional rhythm).** Following an extrasystole (2d beat, possibly atrial with P hidden within the preceding T), junctional rhythm gets a chance to start in the compensatory pause. It continues, but there must be retrograde block to the atria, as the antegrade sinus P waves catch up with the junctional beats (*antegrade* P preceding QRS in beat no. 7) and then take over the rhythm (last two beats). In the period with junctional rhythm there thus is atrioventricular dissociation. Note that the antegrade P waves are negative (M lead) and that the junctional beats (nos. 3-7) have a slightly aberrant shape.

111

133

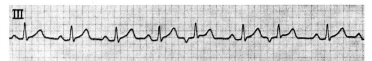

134

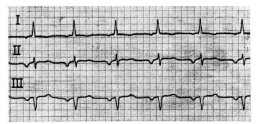

135*

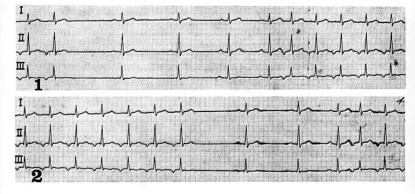

CORONARY SINUS RHYTHMS

This term is used for single beats and rhythms that are characterized by the P waves having the same "retrograde" shape as in junctional rhythm, but the P-R interval is normal or at any rate > 0.12 second. Recent studies, however, suggest that a number of these rhythms do not originate from the region at the entrance of the coronary sinus in the right atrium but originate from ectopic centers in the left atrium. It is not certain whether also some of those rhythms, which, according to current criteria, are called junctional (see p. 111), are left atrial rhythms.

133 Supraventricular extrasystoles of coronary sinus type. This involves beats nos. 5 and 7, which are extrasystoles (arriving prematurely) and have P waves of retrograde shape with a P-R interval that is only slightly shorter (0.16-0.17 second) than the P-R interval of the sinus beats (0.18-0.20 second).

134 Coronary sinus rhythm. The P waves are of retrograde shape, but the P-R interval is 0.14-0.16 second; in other words, normal, so that the rhythm originates above the atrioventricular junction. QRS shows left axis deviation but hardly LAH, as Q is missing in I (cf. p. 55).

135 Repetitive supraventricular tachycardia of coronary sinus type. Continuous strips 1 and 2. The periods with tachycardia (first two and last five beats in strip 1 and first seven and last two beats in strip 2) show retrograde type P waves with P-R interval of 0.16 second. Here we have periods with sinus rhythm for comparison, and can see that the P waves are, generally speaking, in the opposite direction to those from the sinoatrial node, and that the P-R interval is, practically speaking, the same in the sinus beats and in the ectopic beats. Note that the tachycardia periods cannot be junctional with retrograde P (and prolonged retrograde conduction), since they *commence* with aberrant P waves.

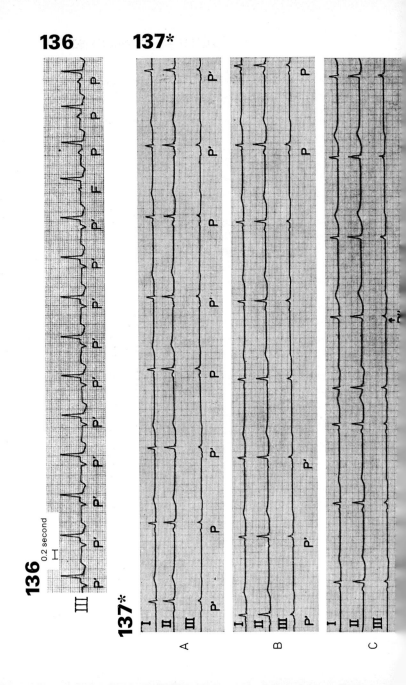

136

0.2 second

III

P' P' P' P' P' P' P' P' P' P' F P P

137*

A

I
II
III

P' P P P' P' P' P

B

I
II
III

P' P' P' P P

C

I
II
III

WANDERING PACEMAKER

By wandering pacemaker is understood a state in which the pacemaker of the heart changes place within the region sinoatrial node, atria and atrioventricular junction, and in which atria and ventricles in the single beat are activated from the same focus (in contrast to atrioventricular dissociation; see p. 133).

The pacemaker can wander: (1) In the sinoatrial node: the shape of the P wave changes from beat to beat without any change in the P-R interval. Can be confused with respiratory changes in the P waves. (2) In the atria: the P wave changes shape at the same time as a change in the P-R interval. (3) Between sinoatrial node and atrioventricular junction: P and P-R change from sinus rhythm to junctional rhythm criteria. (4) In the atrioventricular junction: junctional rhythm, where the relation of P wave to QRS changes.

The change in the pacemaker not uncommonly is precipitated by an extrasystole.

136 **Wandering pacemaker.** The first part of the curve shows retrograde P waves (P') and P-R = 0.19 second: coronary sinus rhythm. The last three beats show antegrade P waves (P), P-R = 0.21 second and slightly more rapid rate: sinus rhythm. One P wave (marked F) can be an atrial fusion beat (simultaneous depolarization of the atria from the two centers). Note the time marking.

137 **Wandering pacemaker.** Patient with bradycardia. Selected strips within minutes. (A) A change is seen between upright P (marked P) and wider, diphasic P (P') with simultaneous change in the P-R interval. This probably is a case of wandering pacemaker in the atria, as P' does not have an obvious "junctional" shape and has P-R < 0.12 second. (B) Here, a gradual shift is seen from one pacemaker to the other. P and P-R intervals in beats nos. 4, 5 and 6 show transitional shape between P and P'. (C) After an atrial extrasystole (beat no. 4), the pacemaker changes to junctional rhythm. The negative "junctional" P wave is seen just preceding QRS in beat no. 5 (P''), but hidden within QRS in the last three beats: wandering pacemaker between sinoatrial node and atrioventricular junction following an extrasystole.

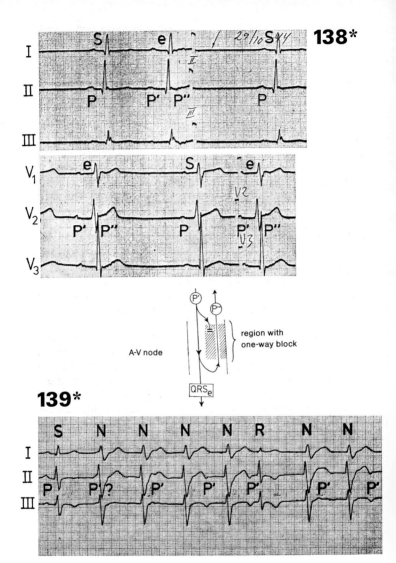

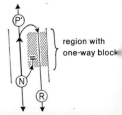

This rare arrhythmia is included in the atlas to illustrate that extrasystole-like beats can be due alone to disturbances of conduction and need not presuppose increased excitability of an ectopic focus. Reciprocal beats (syn.: echo beats, return beats, "return extrasystoles") are beats that arise when an impulse, after having passed the atrioventricular node one way, then turns back to ("re-enters") the chamber from which it originated, so delayed that it once more can depolarize this chamber (but before the next beat in the basic rhythm). It is a condition that there are parallel routes through the atrioventricular node and that one of these routes has one-way block.

138 **Atrial reciprocal beats.** The beats marked e are atrial extra-systoles: they have ectopic (atrial) P waves (P') and a longer P-R interval than the sinus beats (marked S). The QRS complexes of the extra-systoles are followed by P waves (P'') of retrograde shape. P'' are atrial echo beats, and the route of the impulse is shown schematically below the recordings: from the atria to the atrioventricular node and from there simultaneously to ventricles and back to the atria.

139 **Ventricular reciprocal beats.** The first beat is a sinus beat (S); the next beats constitute an accelerated junctional rhythm with aberrant QRS complexes (bundle branch block patterns, marked N). The junctional QRS complexes are followed by P waves of retrograde (inverted) shape (P'). The retrograde conduction time ("R-P' interval") is increasing ("reverse Wenckebach period") and finally becomes so long that the impulse once again can be conducted antegrade after having reached up to the atria. The QRS complex R thus is a ventricular reciprocal beat. It is characterized by the fact that (1) the shape resembles that of the sinus beat, (2) it is preceded by a retrograde P wave and (3) it is premature and blocks the next idiojunctional beat. It can be seen that the differential diagnosis with respect to an atrial (in particular, coronary sinus) extrasystole is difficult. The sketch below the recording shows the probable route of the impulse.

140

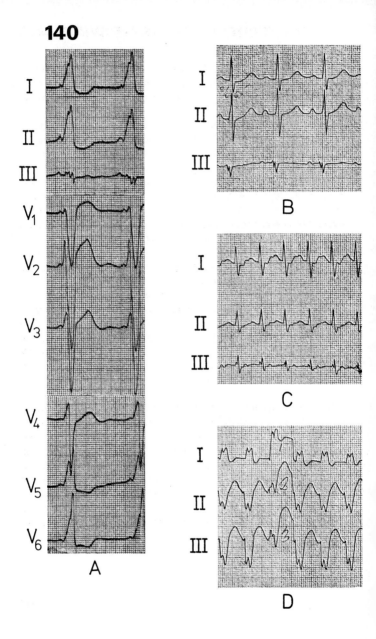

PRE-EXCITATION AND W-P-W SYNDROME 1

By pre-excitation is understood a state in which sinus impulses activate the ventricles abnormally early: the P waves are of normal ("sinus rhythm") shape, but the P-R interval is abnormally short, ≤ 0.11 second. There are two main types:

Simple pre-excitation = nodal bypass, presumably due to an abnormally rapid conduction through fibers from the atrium to the upper part of the bundle of His ("James' bundle"). The QRS complexes are normal.

W-P-W syndrome (Wolff-Parkinson-White syndrome), probably due to the ventricular activation commencing prematurely via abnormal fibers between one of the atria and one of the ventricles ("Kent's bundle") or between the bundle of His and the ventricular myocardium ("Mahaim's fibers"). The remainder of the ventricular activation takes place normally. QRS becomes abnormally wide, consisting of an early part ("delta wave") and a normal final part. Often, a bend or notch is seen in QRS between the two parts.

Subjects with W-P-W syndrome often have a tendency to *attacks of supraventricular tachycardia,* presumably because of the formation of a circus movement, using as one pathway the abnormal fibers ("re-entry phenomenon"). During tachycardia, QRS can be of narrow supraventricular type or wide and aberrant. If atrial fibrillation occurs in W-P-W syndrome, the ventricular response usually is very rapid and with aberrant ventricular conduction.

140 Intermittent W-P-W syndrome with attacks of tachycardia in a 9-month-old infant. (A) There are positive P waves with short P-R interval and wide QRS complexes, in which large delta waves are clearly seen (hatched to the right in V_6): W-P-W syndrome. (B) Some days later, normal electrocardiogram. (C) Attack of supraventricular tachycardia. The P waves are clearly seen, partly superimposed on the T waves. (D) Attack of supraventricular tachycardia with aberrant conduction (wide complexes). The P waves cannot be seen, so that this recording alone does not permit a differential diagnosis with respect to ventricular tachycardia.

141

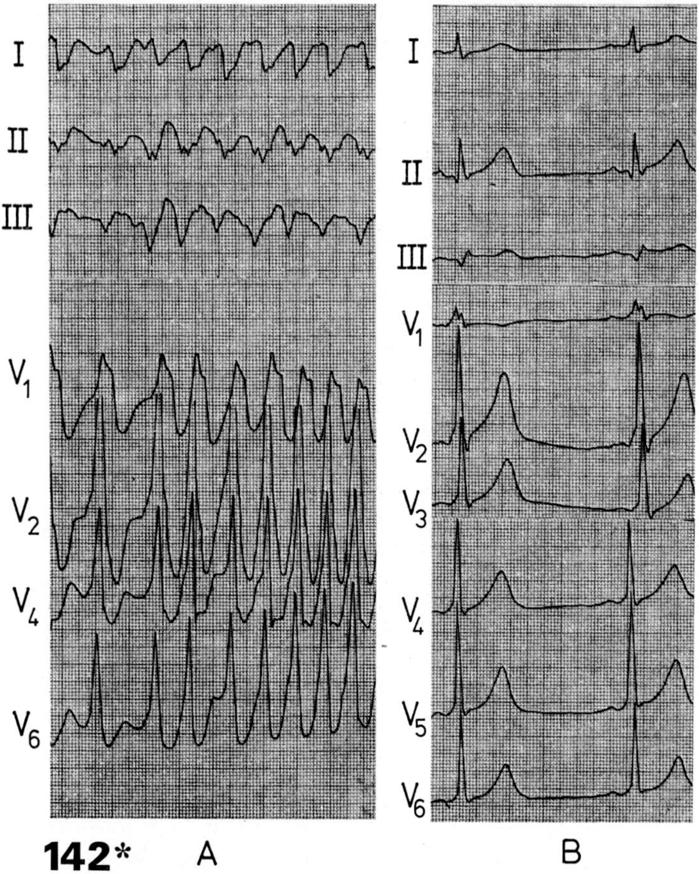
I
II
III
V1
V2
V4
V6
I
II
III
V1
V2
V3
V4
V5
V6
A
B

142*

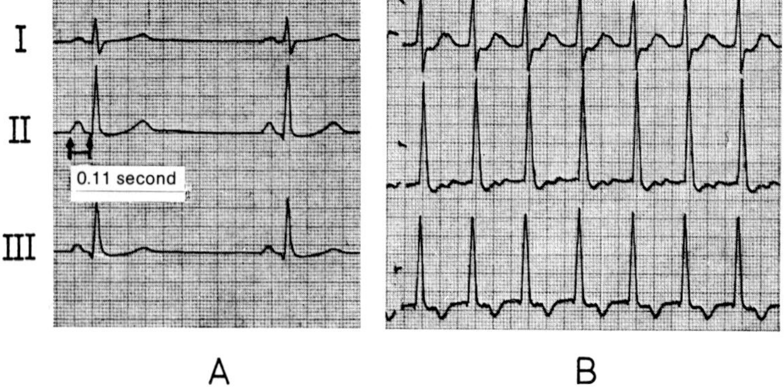
I
II
0.11 second
III
A
B

141 W-P-W syndrome with "pseudoventricular tachycardia".
18-year-old man. (A) On admission, rapid irregular tachycardia is seen
with wide, bizarre QRS complexes. The rate is, on the average, about
275/min. The rhythm is so irregular and fast that atrial fibrillation is
highly probable. Tachycardias such as this can, in the acute stage, be
difficult to distinguish from ventricular tachycardia or ventricular flutter.
(B) On the next day, spontaneous regression is seen to sinus rhythm.
W-P-W syndrome is seen with obvious delta waves (e.g., in V₂). Some
authors distinguish between W-P-W syndrome type A with positive
main deflection in V_1 and type B with negative main deflection in V_1.
According to this classification, **140,** page 118, represents type B and
the present figure type A.

142 Pre-excitation with supraventricular tachycardia. Child with
repeated attacks of palpitation. (A) Between attacks, the electrocardiogram is normal, apart from slightly shortened P-R interval = 0.11 second.
(B) During attack, supraventricular tachycardia is seen. The P waves
are seen clearly, QRS is of narrow supraventricular type. The rate is
about 200/min. Such cases of simple pre-excitation with supraventricular paroxysmal tachycardia often are called Lown-Ganong-Levine
syndrome. The mechanism of tachycardia is considered analogous to
that in W-P-W syndrome.

143

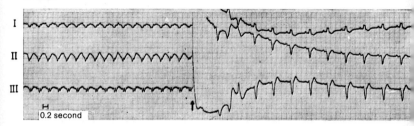

I

II

III

0.2 second

144

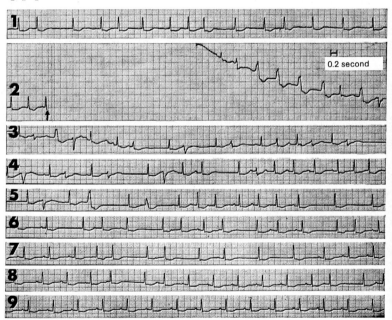

1

2

0.2 second

3

4

5

6

7

8

9

CARDIOVERSION

Hereby is understood treatment of ectopic rhythms with an apparatus that, with the aid of the patient's own R wave, can trigger off a brief D.C. shock at a predetermined point in the heart cycle outside the "vulnerable period".

143 **Treatment of ventricular tachycardia.** The rate of the tachycardia is about 160/min. The D.C. shock is applied at the arrow and for a moment displaces the electrocardiogram. When this again becomes visible, there is sinus rhythm after an extrasystole, rate about 80/min. The patient had myocardial infarction, but this is not seen in the electrocardiogram, as there is left bundle branch block.

144 **Treatment of atrial fibrillation.** Sinus rhythm also often appears here immediately or after a short period with extrasystoles; but in this patient there were disturbances of rhythm long after the D.C. shock, so that the illustration shows a very long course. The curve strips 1-9 follow each other chronologically. All strips show lead II.

Curve 1:   Atrial fibrillation with controlled ventricular response. Digitalis effect on S-T segment and T wave.

Curve 2:   D.C. shock at the arrow. When the electrocardiogram returns, a single sinus beat is seen, and then many ventricular extrasystoles.

Curve 3:   Still many ventricular extrasystoles from various foci, in periods coupled. A single pause (sinoatrial block) with a junctional escape beat.

Curve 4:   In addition to ventricular extrasystoles, a few pauses are seen followed by junctional escape beats and finally by two atrial extrasystoles.

Curve 5:   To the left, junctional beats with coupled ventricular extrasystoles; in the middle, sinus rhythm with atrial extrasystoles, to the right, junctional rhythm.

Curves 6-8: Sinus rhythm, although occasionally pauses still appear (sinoatrial block), after which there are single or a couple of junctional escape beats.

Curve 9:   Sinus rhythm.

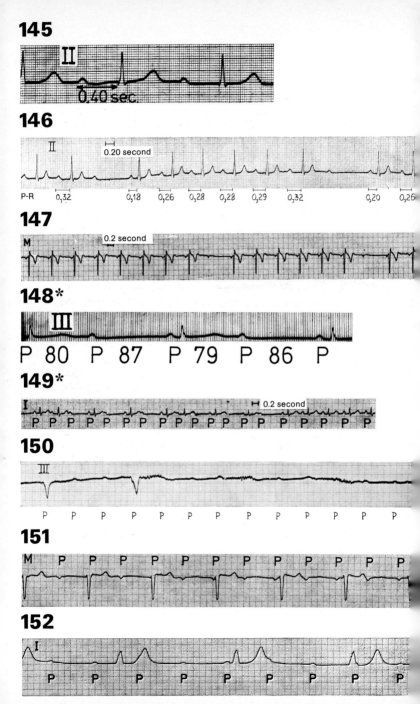

145

II

0.40 sec.

146

II

0.20 second

P-R 0,32 0,18 0,26 0,28 0,28 0,29 0,32 0,20 0,26

147

M

0.2 second

148*

III

P 80 P 87 P 79 P 86 P

149*

I

0.2 second

P P P P P P P P P P P P P P P P P P P P

150

III

P P P P P P P P P P P P P

151

M P P P P P P P P P P P

152

I

P P P P P P P P P

ATRIOVENTRICULAR BLOCK

First degree: Prolonged P-R interval, all beats conducted.

Second degree: Some beats are not conducted. Three types: *Mobitz type I* = Wenckebach. *Mobitz type II:* Without preceding change in the P-R interval, one or several ventricular beats are "dropped". *Block with 2:1 atrioventricular response.*

Third degree: No beat conducted.

First degree + second degree = incomplete, third degree = complete block.

145 **First degree atrioventricular block.** Prolonged P-R interval.

146 **Second degree atrioventricular block, Mobitz type I.** Wenckebach periods: After a period with gradually increasing P-R interval, a QRST is dropped, after which there again is increasing P-R interval, etc. In this case, it has resulted in 7:6 block.

147 **Second degree atrioventricular block, Mobitz type II.** At two points, the P waves are not conducted to the ventricles without the P-R interval having changed in the preceding beats. There are dropped ventricular beats "without prior warning".

148 **Second degree atrioventricular block, 2:1 block.** Every second atrial impulse is conducted, and with normal P-R interval. In addition, there can be seen the so-called *ventriculo-phasic sinus arrhythmia* (the cause of which is obscure). Those P-P intervals that contain QRS complexes are slightly shorter than the others (times in hundreths of a second).

149 **Varying second degree atrioventricular block.** The P waves nos. 1-2-3 and nos. 8-9-10 are conducted with short Wenckebach periods with 3:2 block. The P waves nos. 4-5-6-7 and nos. 11-12-13-14 are conducted only with 2:1 atrioventricular response and show ventriculophasic sinus arrhythmia. The block is terminated from P wave no. 15.

150 **Third degree atrioventricular block with transition to ventricular asystole.** The P waves continue, but the ventricular rhythm ceases. This results in Adams-Stokes attack or death, depending on whether the ventricular action is reinstituted or not.

151 **Third degree atrioventricular block.** Independent P and QRS rhythm, here a junctional rhythm, rate 58/min.

152 **Third degree atrioventricular block.** As **151,** but QRS is idioventricular, 32/min. Often a more serious type than **151.**

153

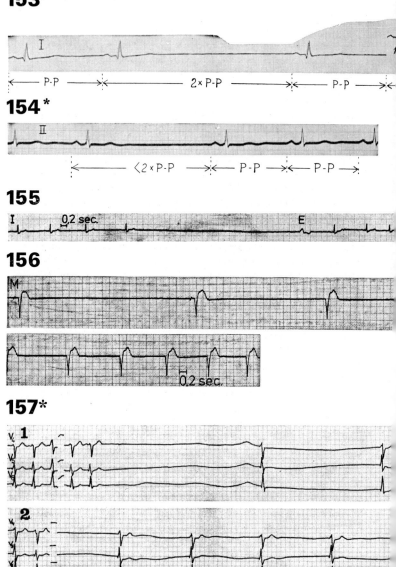

I

$\longleftarrow$ P-P $\longrightarrow$ $\longleftarrow$ 2×P-P $\longrightarrow$ $\longleftarrow$ P-P $\longrightarrow$

154 *

II

$\longleftarrow$ <2×P-P $\longrightarrow$ $\longleftarrow$ P-P $\longrightarrow$ $\longleftarrow$ P-P $\longrightarrow$

155

I 0.2 sec. E

156

M

0.2 sec.

157*

1

2

SINOATRIAL BLOCK

By analogy with atrioventricular block, it is considered that three degrees of exit block can be found from the sinoatrial node to the atria. Since the activity of the sinoatrial node itself cannot be seen in the electrocardiogram, first degree block (prolonged conduction time) therefore cannot be recognized.

Second degree block of the Wenckebach type exists, but the diagnosis is for advanced students. Incomplete block, in analogy with Mobitz II atrioventricular block, presents by one or several heartbeats being dropped. *Third degree sinoatrial block* cannot be distinguished in the electrocardiogram from nonfunction of the sinoatrial node (sinus arrest). Here, the heart either stops beating (cardiac arrest) or an escape rhythm comes into function (see pp. 107 and 111-113). The designation "sick sinus syndrome", tachy-bradycardia syndrome, is used for conditions in which atrial tachycardia alternates with severe depression of sinoatrial node function.

153 **Second degree sinoatrial block.** A complete P-QRS-T complex has dropped out. The pause is exactly the double of the basic P-P duration; this is described as a "dropped beat". Compare this with the atrioventricular Mobitz II block **147,** page 125.

154 **Second degree sinoatrial block.** A P-QRS-T complex of normal shape appears too late. The pause is < 2 × P-P. (May be a sinoatrial exit block with Wenckebach phenomenon, as the last P-P interval is shorter than the next to last; see textbooks.)

155 **Third degree sinoatrial block or sinus arrest.** After four beats with sinus bradycardia (45-50/min), electrical standstill develops, which is "rescued" by a ventricular escape beat (E), after which sinus rhythm develops. Patient with carotid sinus syndrome.

156 **Severe sinoatrial block or sinus arrest** (continuous recording). First two sinus beats, showing severe sinoatrial block, as their mutual distance corresponds to a rate of 11-12/min. Then third degree sinoatrial block, which is "rescued" by a junctional escape rhythm. Note that this only gradually speeds up.

157 **"Sick sinus syndrome".** About 20 seconds between curves 1 and 2. Two runs of supraventricular (presumably atrial) tachycardia, alternating with sinus arrest, junctional escape beats and junctional rhythm.

158

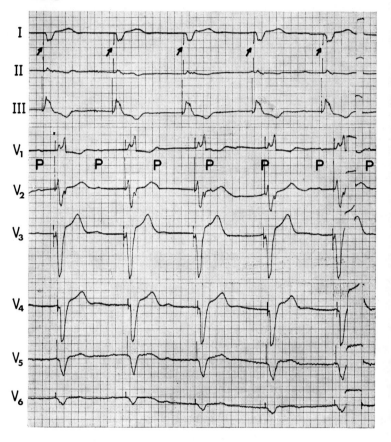

ARTIFICIAL PACEMAKER RHYTHMS 1

Artificial pacemakers have been employed increasingly in the treatment of patients with Adams-Stokes attacks and certain other patients with bradyarrhythmias.

Pacemaker impulses are of few volts and last 0.5-2 milliseconds. In the electrocardiogram, therefore, they are seen as very narrow vertical lines of "almost no duration" but with an amplitude of one half to several mV. However, it is important to remember that some electrocardiographic recorders have such inertia that the pacemaker impulses remain small, making interpretation difficult. In the interpretation, it is of importance to know the type of pacemaker.

A *fixed-rate pacemaker* (asynchronous, competitive) sends out impulses all the time. A *demand pacemaker* (noncompetitive) will only depolarize the myocardium when a pause of a certain length appears in a patient's inherent rhythm. *QRS-inhibited demand pacemakers* (ventricular-inhibited) will be inhibited by the patient's own QRS complexes. As long as there is no pause in the patient's inherent rhythm, no pacemaker impulses are seen in the electrocardiogram. With pauses longer than a previously determined size ("escape interval"), the pacemaker impulses start with an inherent rate that is also fixed in advance. *QRS-triggered demand pacemakers* (ventricular synchronous) will be triggered by the patient's own QRS complexes. Even though there are no pauses in the patient's inherent rhythm, pacing signals are seen in the middle of the patient's own QRS complexes but do not stimulate contraction, the ventricle being refractory. With pauses longer than a predetermined duration ("escape interval"), the pacemaker transmits its own impulses with an inherent rate that is determined in advance. The seldom-used *P-triggered demand pacemakers* (atrial synchronous) are triggered by the patient's P waves.

158 **Fixed-rate pacemaker rhythm.** The pacemaker impulses are indicated by arrows in lead I. The patient had third degree atrioventricular block, and his own idioventricular rhythm was permanently depressed by the pacemaker rhythm, which therefore controlled the ventricles with a rate of 63/min. The pacemaker electrodes were implanted in the wall of the left ventricle (right bundle branch block pattern). Today, pacing usually is carried out through electrodes transvenously inserted into the right ventricle, giving left bundle branch block patterns **(159-162).**

159

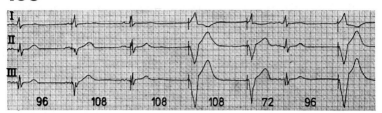

96 108 108 108 72 96

160

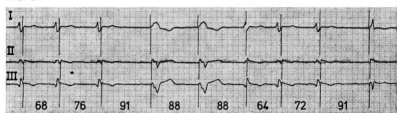

68 76 91 88 88 64 72 91

161

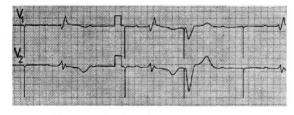

162*

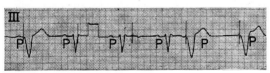

ARTIFICIAL PACEMAKER RHYTHMS 2

159 QRS-inhibited demand pacemaker. The first beat is a sinus beat. As a result of sinus bradycardia, the pacemaker manages to give off impulses, so that the pacemaker and the sinoatrial node together depolarize the ventricles in beats nos. 2 and 3, which thus are fusion beats. The sinus bradycardia now becomes so pronounced that the pacemaker alone initiates beat no. 4. Beat no. 5 once more is a fusion beat, no. 6 is a pure sinus beat and no. 7 is a pure pacemaker beat. The intervals are in hundredths of a second. It is seen that the pacemaker's "escape interval" (R to pace impulse) is 0.96 second, whereas its inherent rate arrives at intervals of 1.08 seconds.

160 QRS-triggered demand pacemaker. Patient with atrial fibrillation and slow ventricular response. The first three beats are the patient's own conducted beats. It is seen that QRS triggers the pacemaker: pace impulses in the middle of QRS. After a pause in the ventricular rhythm of 0.91 second ("escape interval"), the pacemaker takes over the depolarization of the ventricles (beats nos. 4 and 5) with a rate of 68/sec. Beats nos. 6 and 9 are fusion beats, as the pacemaker is depolarizing the ventricles at the very moment a beat is conducted from the atria. Beats nos. 7 and 8 are conducted from the atria (shape as in the first three).

161 Pacemaker malfunction. QRS-inhibited demand pacemaker. Two faults are seen: First, pacemaker impulses nos. 1, 2 and 4 do not initiate ventricular beats, even though they occur outside the refractory period of the ventricles; only beat no. 3 is a pacemaker-induced beat, perhaps because it falls within the supernormal phase; see page 29. In the second place, the pacemaker is not inhibited properly by the patient's own beats: own beat no. 1 inhibits but no. 2 does not.

162 Pacemaker malfunction. QRS-inhibited demand pacemaker implanted in patient with intermittent atrioventricular block. The curve shows the patient in a phase with sinus rhythm (P waves). The demand function of the pacemaker is seen to fail: it does not "sense" the patient's own QRS complexes (QRS nos. 2, 3 and 4), and therefore *continues to operate as a fixed-rate pacemaker.* On the other hand, it paces well enough, as it initiates QRS each time the pacing impulses fall outside the refractory period (QRS nos. 1, 5 and 6).

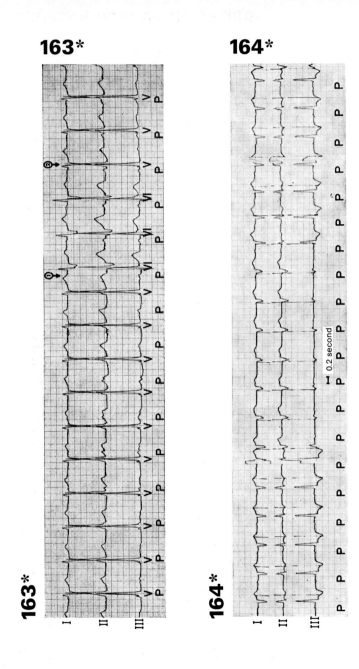

ATRIOVENTRICULAR DISSOCIATION

Atrioventricular dissociation in the broadest sense designates the *phenomenon that atria and ventricles are activated by separate centers.* It occurs (1) with third degree atrioventricular block, (2) temporarily in various dysrhythmias, e.g., ventricular extrasystoles and parasystole, (3) for longer periods frequently in ventricular tachycardia and (4) in conditions where the rate of an idiojunctional or idioventricular rhythm is close to the sinus rate while at the same time there is retrograde block but not antegrade block via the atrioventricular node ("isorhythmic dissociation").

Atrioventricular dissociation in the narrowest sense comprises only (4). It occurs in periods of retardation of the sinus rate and/or acceleration of the rate of the ectopic focus. The following are the main types: Sinus bradycardia with periodic junctional escape rhythm, **10,** page 38. Sinus bradycardia with accelerated idioventricular rhythm, **120,** page 107. Accelerated idiojunctional rhythm, **163,** below. Pacemaker-induced cases, **164,** below.

163

163 **Atrioventricular dissociation with interference.** There is "accelerated idiojunctional rhythm" with rate 111/min, which controls the ventricles (marked V), whereas the sinoatrial node (P) beats slightly more slowly, about 106/min. In the left part of the curve, P and V beat independently of each other: the P rhythm is not inhibited by the V rhythm, as there is retrograde block to the atria. At ①, P arrives so late after V that the impulse reaches the ventricles outside the refractory period, so that there now is conduction of three beats. At ②, the V rhythm again anticipates a conducted P rhythm. This is interference in the classic sense of the word (see p. 27), as the conducted beats (ventricular capture beats V-I) interfere with the V rhythm. The third V-I beat is a fusion beat.

164

164 **"Artificial" atrioventricular dissociation with interference.** Implanted fixed-rate pacemaker. There is, at the time of recording, no antegrade atrioventricular block, since the P waves can conduct, provided that the impulses reach the ventricles outside the refractory period. On the other hand, there must be retrograde block, as the P waves continue independently of the pacemaker rhythm. Here, this is only slightly slower than the rate of the sinoatrial node. The middle strip of the curve shows atrioventricular dissociation. In the left and right part, the sinus beats are conducted, so they "interfere" with the pacemaker rhythm, as the pacemaker impulses here occur in the refractory period of the ventricle.

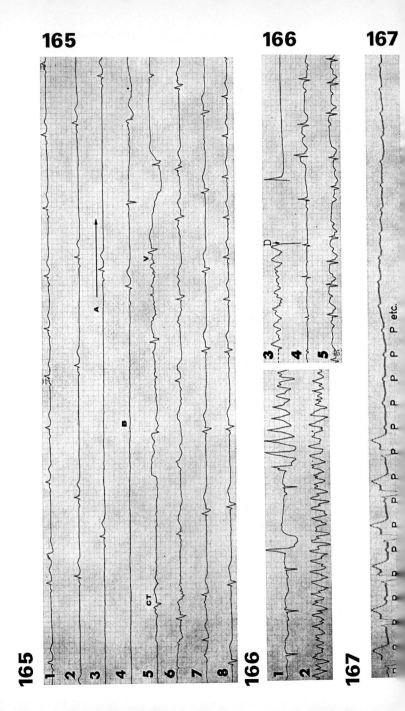

165

1
2
3
4
5
6
7
8

A

B

V

cT

166

1
2
3
4
5

D

167

P P P P P P P P etc.

Clinical *cardiac arrest despite continued electrocardiographic ventricular activity* may be due to a number of causes; e.g., rupture of the heart, rupture of aneurysm of the aorta, large pulmonary emboli.

Cardiac arrest in connection with electrical failure of the ventricular function is of three main types, all shown elsewhere in the atlas but collected here for clarity: (1) *Asystole* because of severe sinoatrial block or sinus arrest. (2) *Ventricular fibrillation.* (3) *Ventricular asystole* with continued atrial activity.

165

166

167

165 **Cardiac arrest – asystole.** Monitoring lead, continuous strips 1-8: (1) Sinus bradycardia and sinus arrhythmia; a ventricular extrasystole (3d beat). (2-3) Increasing bradycardia, increasing to periods with severe (third degree) sinoatrial block or sinus arrest. At A, atropine is given 0.5 mg IV. (4) At B, the patient is unconscious. An ectopic atrial beat is seen, followed by a junctional and a ventricular escape beat. (5) At CT, some "chest thumps" are started, giving an irregular baseline. A response is obtained immediately, but with bradycardia. At V, the patient again is conscious. (6) The chest thumps are continued to the middle of the curve. (7-8) After a period with junctional escape rhythm, there once more is sinus rhythm.

166 **Cardiac arrest – ventricular fibrillation.** Monitoring leads, continuous strips 1-5, although about 1 minute between strips 2 and 3: (1) After three sinus beats, a ventricular extrasystole is seen of "R on T type". After a further sinus beat, a new "R on T" extrasystole starts ventricular flutter, which immediately changes to ventricular fibrillation of the "coarse" type. (2-3) Ventricular fibrillation continues for more than 1 minute, after which at D electrical defibrillation is carried out. After a period with asystole, the activity returns (4), in the beginning with supraventricular arrhythmia of uncertain type, and at the end of (5) sinus rhythm with aberrant ventricular conduction (compare with strip 1) and with atrial extrasystoles.

167 **Cardiac arrest – ventricular asystole.** Monitoring lead. To the left, third degree atrioventricular block is seen with idioventricular rhythm, then ventricular arrest, while the atrial activity continues (P).

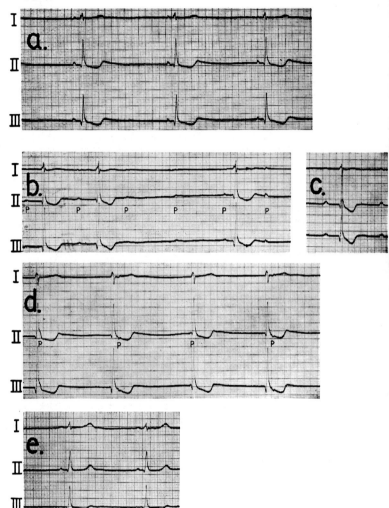

The most frequent *effects of digitalis* on the electrocardiogram are:
(1) A *depression of the S-T segment,* which involves the first of the T wave and is most pronounced at the transition between the S-T segment and the T wave. The changes usually are most pronounced in those leads where the main deflection of QRS is upward.
(2) *Shortening of the Q-T interval* (duration of systole).
These effects are *not* signs of toxic effect of digitalis.

In *digitalis toxicity,* many types of electrocardiographic changes can be seen, among which the most frequent are sinus *bradycardia,* ventricular *extrasystoles,* frequently *coupled extrasystoles* and incomplete *atrioventricular block.* More rare are third degree atrioventricular block, sinoatrial block, junctional rhythm, atrial extrasystoles and paroxysmal atrial tachycardia with atrioventricular block. Severe digitalis intoxication – especially in pre-existing myocardial disease – can result in ventricular tachycardia with danger of death in ventricular fibrillation.

168 **Digitalis poisoning.** A 15-year-old girl has taken 100 digitalis leaf tablets in a suicide attempt. Five minutes later there is vomiting and an unknown number of tablets are brought up.

(a) About 8 hours after taking the tablets. Sinus bradycardia, pronounced S-T changes and shortened Q-T interval.

(b) About 20 hours after taking the tablets. Severe second degree atrioventricular block (the block is varying, on the average 2:1 in the figure).

(c) About 28 hours after taking the tablets. First degree atrioventricular block = prolonged P-R interval (0.25 second).

(d) Four days after taking the tablets. Wandering pacemaker in the atrioventricular junction: P waves of retrograde shape in varying relation to the QRS complexes. As in (b) and (c), still pronounced S-T changes and rather short Q-T interval.

(e) Three weeks after taking the tablets. The electrocardiogram now is within normal range (P-R interval a little short).

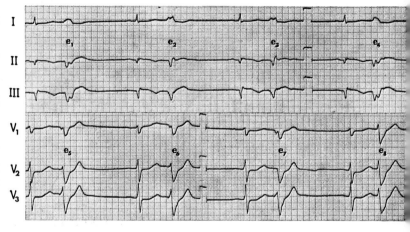

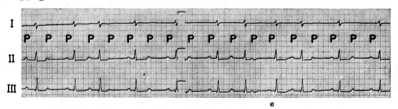

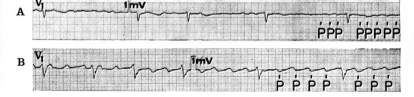

DIGITALIS 2

169 **Digitalis intoxication.** Patient with congestive heart failure following inferior infarction shows signs of intoxication during digoxin treatment, in the form of coupled ventricular extrasystoles (e), which have slightly different shape: In leads I-III, the extrasystoles e_2 and e_3 resemble each other, while e_1 and e_4 are almost identical; in V_{1-3}, e_5, e_6 and e_7 are identical and different from e_8.

170 **Digitalis intoxication.** The P waves show an *atrial tachycardia* with a mean rate of 150/min. There is *second degree atrioventricular block,* varying between 2:1 block and short Wenckebach periods with 3:2 block. The rhythm is further complicated by the beat marked e, which is either an atrial extrasystole or one of the patient's normal sinus beats (note that the P wave of the e beat is premature).

QUINIDINE

The most frequent effects of quinidine on the electrocardiogram are (1) an *increase in width of the QRS complex* and the Q-T interval, (2) a *slower atrial rhythm,* seen particularly in atrial fibrillation and atrial flutter and (3) *in atrial fibrillation and atrial flutter, often a more rapid ventricular response.* Toxic effects can result in a number of changes and risk of asystole or ventricular fibrillation: electrocardiographic monitoring during acute treatment with large doses!

171 **Quinidine effect in atrial fibrillation.** (A) A patient with atrial fibrillation and slow ventricular response. The atrial rate is about 460/min, ventricular rate is about 56/min. (B) Electrocardiogram after a total of 2.4 gm quinidine. The characteristic *quinidine effects* are seen: *The atrial rate has dropped* to about 270/min, *ventricular rate has increased* to about 75/min, *the QRS duration has increased* from 0.07 to 0.10 second. Increase of the QRS duration by 50% is considered an indication for withdrawal of the drug.

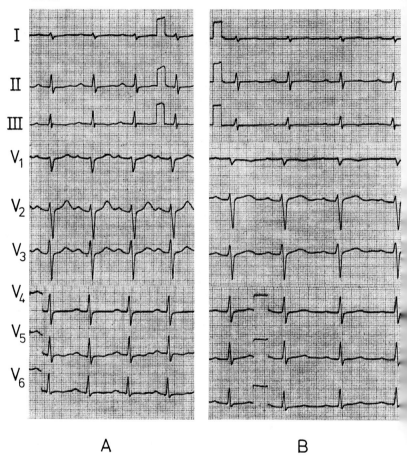

A

B

BETA-ADRENERGIC BLOCKING AGENTS

Apart from their antiarrhythmic effect, beta-blockers show effects on the electrocardiogram that reflect the sympatholytic effect on the heart: (1) The rate of the sinus rhythm becomes slower (negative chronotropic effect). (2) The P-R interval may increase. (3) Larger amplitudes of the T waves may be seen. (4) The Q-T interval can be shortened. It is uncertain whether the last changes are correlated with the negative inotropic effect.

The drugs have been used in an attempt at distinguishing between "functional" changes and ischemic changes (see pp. 59-65) both at rest and during exercise test, since "functional" changes should regress during treatment with beta-blockers. The diagnostic value of such a test still is not clarified.

172 **The effect of beta-blocking agent on the electrocardiogram.** (A) shows an electrocardiogram from a 21-year-old woman with symptoms that suggest neurocirculatory asthenia. A vertical heart position is seen (QRS axis about +90° with small deflections in I), sinus tachycardia 125/min and slight S-T depression with diphasic T in II, III and V_{4-6}. (B) Three-quarters of an hour after administration of 20 mg propranolol orally, a slower sinus rhythm is seen and normalization of the S-T segment and T waves. No change is seen in the P-R interval or the Q-T_c interval.

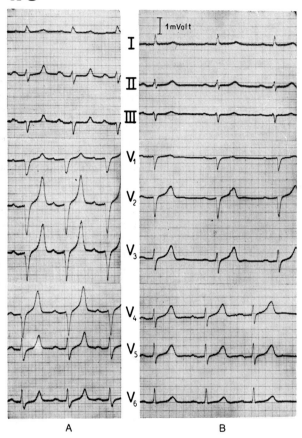

I

II

III

V₁

V₂

V₃

V₄

V₅

V₆

1mVolt

A

B

HYPERPOTASSEMIA

In very severe hyperpotassemia, severe electrocardiographic changes are seen, especially in the form of *atrial arrest* (disappearing P waves) and a ventricular, occasionally irregular rhythm with *wide, bizarre QRS complexes*. The condition can lead to death in ventricular fibrillation or asystole.

In less pronounced degrees of hyperpotassemia there characteristically is an *increase in the amplitude of the T waves* without an increase in width. This often is described as large, "tent-shaped" T waves. High T waves can be seen in the precordial leads in posterior wall infarction (see, for example, **51,** p. 68) and can also be seen normally in young individuals, so that the changes should be followed by series electrocardiography. In addition, decreasing amplitude of the R waves and increasing S waves may be seen.

173 **Hyperpotassemia in uremia and dehydration.** (A) Serum potassium = 7.4 mEq/liter. The characteristic T waves are seen particularly in V_{2-4}. (B) Electrocardiogram after treatment. Serum potassium = 5.0 mEq/liter. The T waves now are normal. In comparison with the hyperpotassemic phase, the QRS duration has also become shorter, and the amplitude of the R waves in the precordial leads has increased and S waves decreased (normalization).

174*

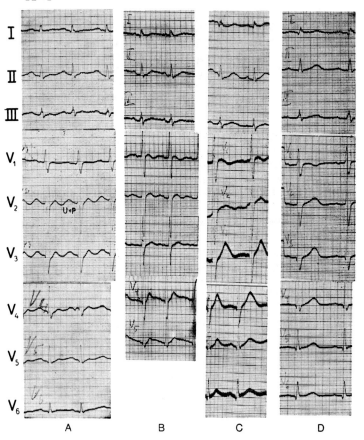

I

II

III

V₁

V₂ U+P

V₃

V₄

V₅

V₆

A   B   C   D

HYPOPOTASSEMIA

Hypopotassemia causes electrocardiographic changes, of which the most characteristic are that *the U wave becomes particularly pronounced.* Previously it was considered that hypopotassemia resulted in a lengthened Q-T interval, but this is because the pronounced U wave was taken to be a T wave. Other electrocardiographic changes in hypopotassemia are *depression of the S-T segment and flat or inverted T Waves.* Dysrhythmias may occur.

174 **Severe hypopotassemia after insulin treatment of diabetic coma.**

(A) Serum potassium = 1.9 mEq/liter. Very pronounced U waves are seen, which coalesce with the following P waves, most clearly in V_{2-3}. The T waves are flat, and there is a tendency to S-T depression; see, for example, II and V_4.

(B) Same day after treatment with intravenous potassium. The U waves are smaller, so there is commencing separation of the U and the P waves (see particularly V_{2-3}). The T waves are larger.

(C) On the next day, serum potassium = 3.0 mEq/liter. Further normalization. The U waves still can be identified as an extra hump on the descending limb of the now large T waves (see, for example, lead II).

(D) Twelve days later. Serum potassium = 4.4 mEq/liter. Now no U waves. S-T segments and T waves are normal.

175

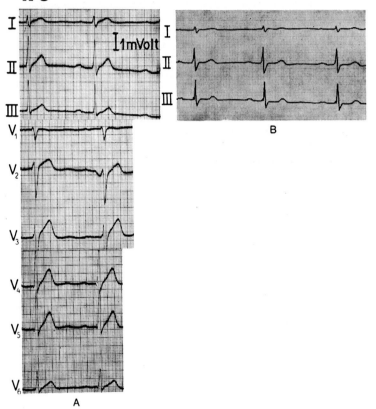

In hypercalcemia, the characteristic change in the electrocardiogram is a *shortening of* the duration of systole, *the Q-T interval.*

175 **Hypercalcemia caused by a malignant tumor in the parathyroid glands.** (A) Serum calcium = 15.7 mg/100 ml (serum phosphorus = 4.7 mg/100 ml and serum potassium = 5.0 mEq/liter). The short Q-T interval is obvious; the T wave follows immediately after the S wave. In addition, there is prolonged P-R interval (0.24 second). (B) The standard limb leads after removal of the primary tumor. Serum calcium = 9.1 mg/100 ml. There now is a well-defined S-T segment and the electrocardiogram is, in general, normal. (On subsequent recurrence, changes again appeared as in A.)

176*

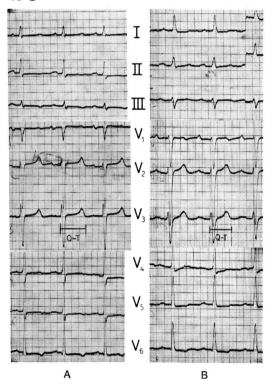

I
II
III
V₁
V₂
V₃
V₄
V₅
V₆

A   B

HYPOCALCEMIA

Hypocalcemia results in a lengthening of the S-T segment, resulting in a *lengthened Q-T interval*. The T wave usually is normal.

For calculation of the corrected Q-T interval Q-T$_c$, see pages 21-22.

176 **Hypocalcemia in a patient with chronic pyelonephritis and uremia.** (A) Serum calcium = 8.2 mg/100 ml (serum potassium = 5.7 mEq/liter). The curves show Q-T$_c$ = Q-T/$\sqrt{R\text{-}R}$ = 0.37/$\sqrt{0.62}$ = 0.47; i.e., the Q-T interval is lengthened.

The curves show further changes due to simultaneous (uremic) pericarditis, the T waves being low to inverted in some leads (see p. 79). (B) After repeated intravenous injections of calcium, Q-T$_c$ = 0.39, i.e., normal (unfortunately, the serum calcium was not checked).

EXERCISES

EXERCISES

(For interpretation, see p. 167)

I

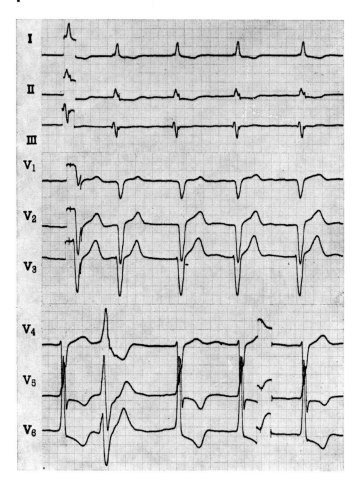

II

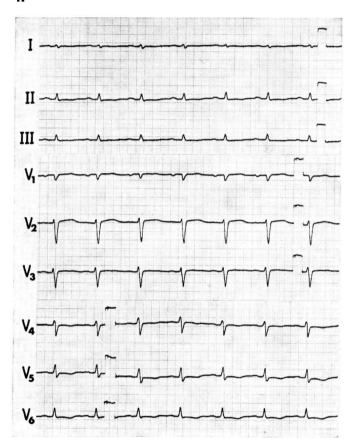

EXERCISES

(For interpretation, see p. 168)

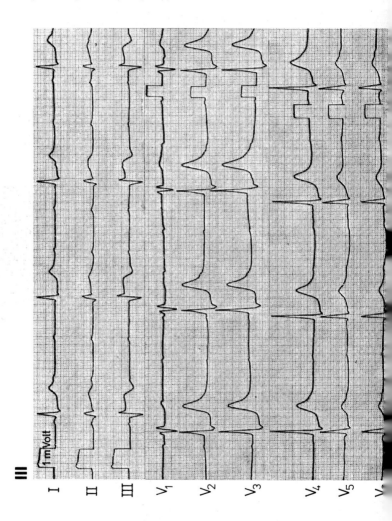

1 mVolt

I   II   III   V$_1$ V$_2$ V$_3$ V$_4$ V$_5$ V

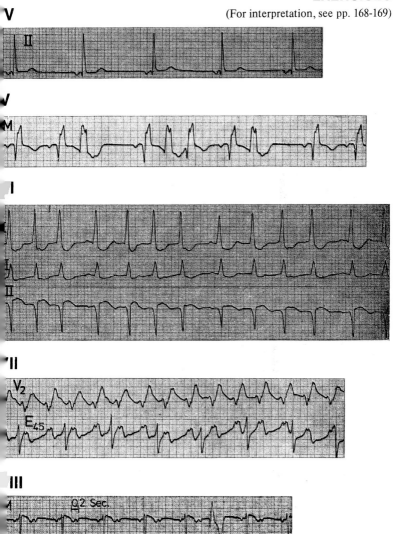

155

EXERCISES

(For interpretation, see p. 169)

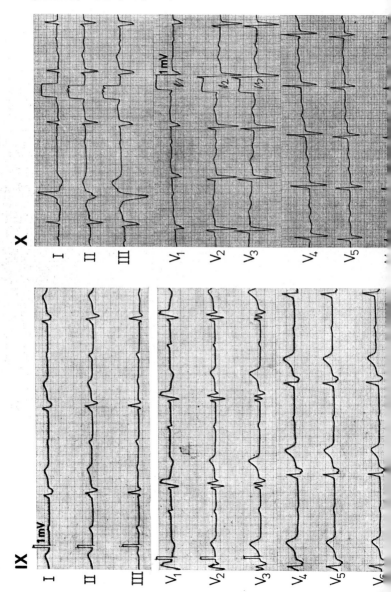

XI

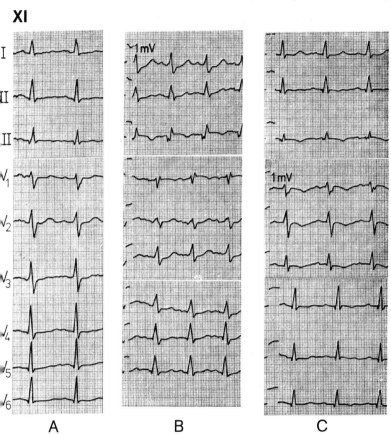

A B C

45-year-old woman with severe obesity, admitted to the surgical depart-
ment on the 6th of November for tumor of the breast and renal calculus.
On the 10th of November, an acute attack with pain in the chest and
tendency to faint. Electrocardiograms: (A) 6th November. (B) 10th
November. (C) 11th November.

EXERCISES

(For interpretation, see p. 170)

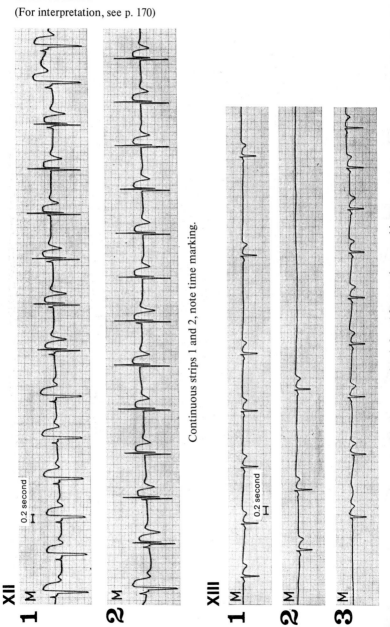

XII
1 M
0.2 second

2 M

Continuous strips 1 and 2, note time marking.

XIII
1 M
0.2 second

2 M

3 M

XIV

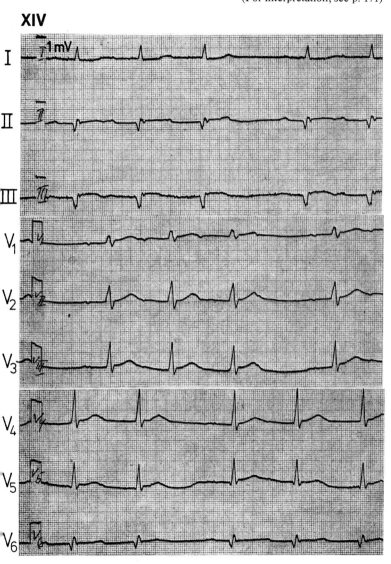

EXERCISES

(For interpretation, see pp. 171-172)

XV

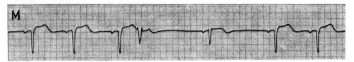

XVI

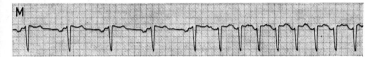

XVII

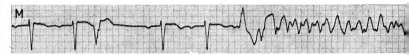

XVIII

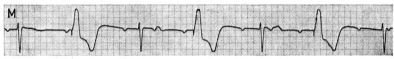

XIX

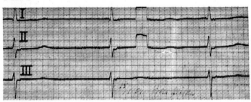

XX

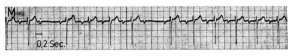

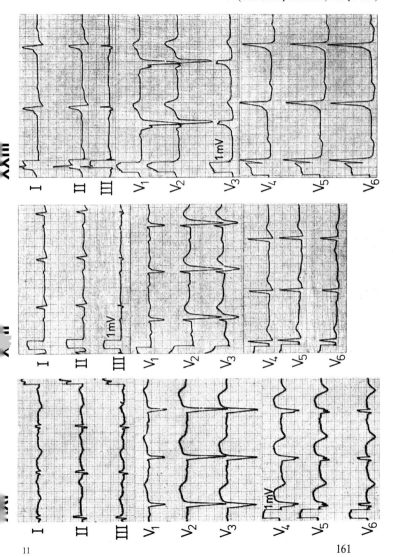

EXERCISES

(For interpretation, see p. 173)

XXIV

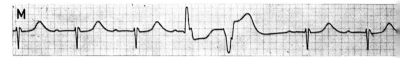

XXV

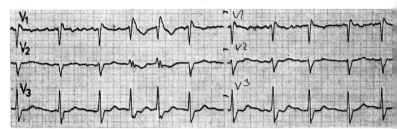

XXVI

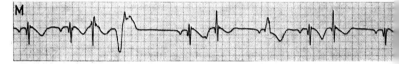

XXVII

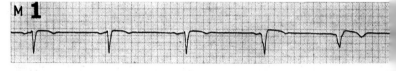

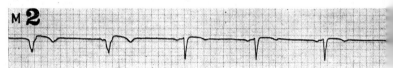

XXVIII

Continuous strips 1 and 2.

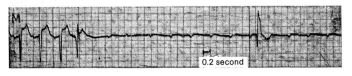

0.2 second

XXIX

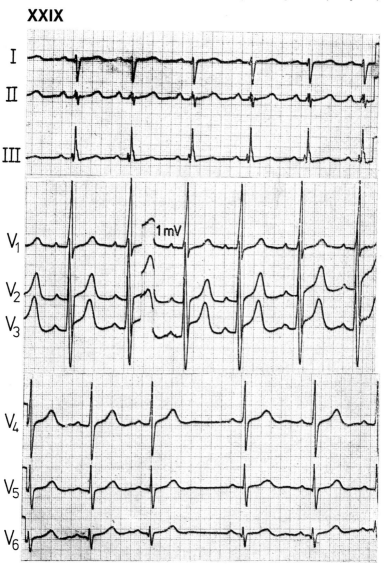

EXERCISES

(For interpretation, see p. 174)

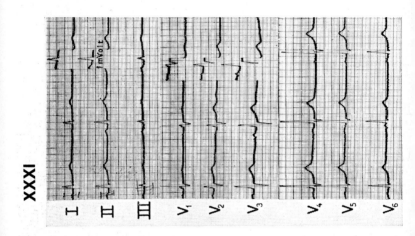

XXXI

I II III V₁ V₂ V₃ V₄ V₅ V₆

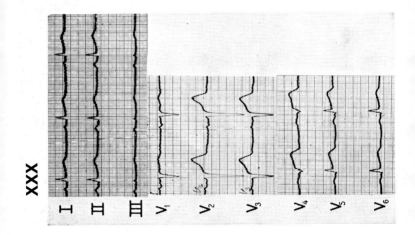

XXX

I II III V₁ V₂ V₃ V₄ V₅ V₆

164

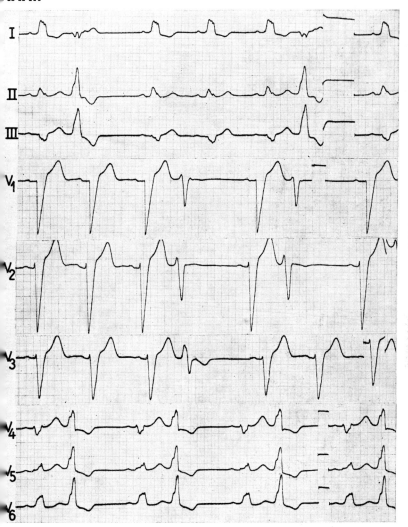

EXERCISES

(For interpretation, see pp. 174-175)

XXXIII

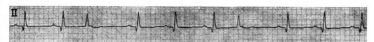

XXXIV

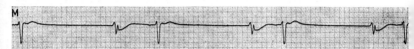

XXXV

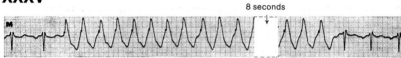

XXXVI

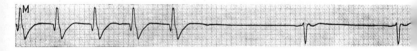

XXXVII

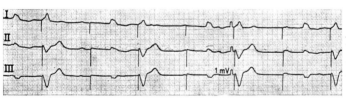

Implanted QRS-inhibited demand pacemaker.

XXXVIII

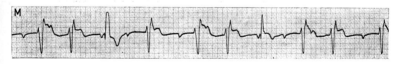

"KEY" TO EXERCISES

In order to illustrate the procedure, a complete analysis is given for the first three exercises along the schematic lines indicated in the introduction, pages 11-22. In the case of the other exercises, only a description of the abnormalities is provided together with the conclusion.

I (1) *Rhythm:* Slightly irregular in basic rhythm. In addition, an early beat in V_{4-6} with increase in width and deviant shape, a ventricular extrasystole. (2) *Rate* in I-III mean value of 87/min. (3) *P waves:* Not seen clearly. In V_{1-2}, toward the end it is possible to glimpse rapid "fibrillation waves". (5) *QRS: Duration:* Normal = 0.11 second (V_3). *Axis:* Normal (the net area in III is negative but numerically less than the area in both I and II). *Configuration:* Abnormal in the precordial leads. There are large QS complexes, but only in V_{1-2}, and the R wave is small in V_3, which together with the very tall R waves in V_{5-6} shows left ventricular hypertrophy (and not myocardial infarction; cf. pp.70-71). (6-7) *The S-T segments and T waves* show pronounced left ventricular strain in the form of depressed S-T and negative T in I, II and V_{5-6}. (8) *U waves:* Normal. (9) *Q-T interval* in the upper normal range; $Q\text{-}T_c = 0.36/\sqrt{0.69} = 0.43$ second.
Conclusion: Pronounced left ventricular hypertrophy and strain without axis deviation. Atrial fibrillation with controlled ventricular response. Ventricular extrasystole.

II (1) *Rhythm:* Regular. (2) *Rate:* 115/min. (3) *P waves:* Normal. (4) *P-R interval:* Normal = 0.14 second. (5) *QRS: Duration:* Normal = 0.08 second. *Axis:* On the boundary between normal axis and right axis deviation. *Configuration:* The shape is normal, but there is pronounced low voltage not only in I-III but also in most of the precordial leads (note the correct 1-mV test throughout). (6) *S-T segments:* Not pathologic. (7) *T waves:* Isoelectric in I, III and V_3 and slightly inverted in II and V_{4-6}. (8) *U waves:* Not seen. (9) *Q-T interval:* Poorly defined but not definitely prolonged, $Q\text{-}T_c = \text{about } 0.30/\sqrt{0.52} = 0.42$ second (V_5).
Conclusion: Pronounced low voltage with low to inverted T waves in several leads. Sinus tachycardia.

167

One may guess at exudative or chronic constrictive pericarditis or severe diffuse myocardial lesions. The electrocardiogram was from a patient with cancer with pericardial effusion.

III (1) *Rhythm:* Regular ventricular rhythm. (2) *Rate:* Ventricular rate = 41/min (bradycardia). (3) *P waves:* There are more P waves than QRS complexes. The P rhythm is almost regular, rate about 110/min, seen best in V₁, where, however, a P wave is hidden within the third QRS complex. The P rhythm is quite independent of the QRS rhythm: Third degree atrioventricular block. (4) *The P-R interval* has no meaning, as there is block. (5) *QRS: Duration* prolonged = 0.12 second. *Configuration:* As in right bundle branch block (double R in V₁), but, in addition, large Q waves in III and also Q in II as in inferior infarction. As a *result* of the infarction pattern, the *axis* becomes slightly left-sided. (6) *S-T segment:* Elevated in III and II and flat depressed in I and V₂₋₅ (as in acute inferior infarction). (7) *T waves:* Diphasic in III, tall and narrow in V₂₋₄. (8) *U waves:* Not seen clearly. (9) *Q-T interval:* Poorly defined = about 0.52, giving Q-T$_c$ = $0.52/\sqrt{1.46}$ = 0.43, i.e., in the upper limit of normal.

Conclusion: Third degree atrioventricular block. The ventricles are controlled either from a center in the left ventricle (cf. text p. 97) or by the atrioventricular junction with simultaneous right bundle branch branch block. Acute inferior myocardial infarction.

IV Regular QRS rhythm of supraventricular (narrow) shape, rate 62/min. QRS preceded by P waves of retrograde shape with P-R interval < 0.12 second.

Conclusion: Junctional rhythm (cf. **129,** p. 111).

V Beats nos. 1, 2, 4, 7, 9 and 10 are sinus beats with QRS of right bundle branch block configuration + large Q waves. Beats nos. 3, 5 and 8 are ventricular extrasystoles of "R on T type", no. 5 is interpolated, as beat no. 6 is conducted, but with slight aberrant ventricular conduction (note the P wave in the T wave of beat no. 5).

Conclusion: "R on T" ventricular extrasystoles (the patient had acute myocardial infarction).

VI QRS complexes show left axis deviation and depressed S-T with low T and short Q-T in I and II (digitalis effect or strain?). The ventricular rhythm is irregular, of the type seen in atrial fibrillation. Closer

168

examination, however, shows P waves with the following distribution:

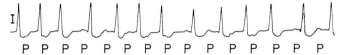

This thus is a case of an atrial tachycardia with second degree atrio-ventricular block in the form of Wenckebach periods, giving 5:4 block; compare **85,** page 91.

Conclusion: Atrial tachycardia with second degree atrioventricular block (patient with digitalis intoxication).

VII   Lead V_2 shows regular tachycardia of uncertain type. Esophageal lead E_{45} shows a rapid ventricular rhythm with broad QRS complexes, rate about 185/min. The P waves (the tall, peaked waves) arrive with slower rate, independent of QRS: Atrioventricular dissociation.

Conclusion: Ventricular tachycardia; compare **110,** page 103.

VIII   An extra P wave is seen superimposed on each T wave; in other words, a P rhythm twice that of QRS. Every second P wave occurs in a fixed relationship to the subequent QRS with P-R = 0.16 second: 2:1 atrioventricular block. At one point, the rhythm is broken, as an extra beat is conducted: QRS no. 6 is conducted with a lengthened P-R and with aberrant ventricular conduction (right bundle branch block pattern). A P wave must be hidden within the T wave of beat no. 6.

Conclusion: Second degree 2:1 atrioventricular block, although at one point 3:2.

IX   The P-R interval is much lengthened = 0.46 second. The sinus rhythm rate 55/min. QRS is increased in width = 0.14 second with configuration as right bundle branch block (rSR' in V_1).

Conclusion: First degree atrioventricular block and right bundle branch block.

X   The P-R interval is lengthened = 0.24-0.26 second. QRS shows pronounced left axis deviation with small initial Q wave in I and R wave in II and III: Left anterior hemiblock (LAH); see page 55. There are no signs of left ventricular hypertrophy in the precordial leads, which are normal apart from S waves right out in V_{5-6}. Beat no. 2 in I-III is a ventricular extrasystole.

169

Conclusion: First degree atrioventricular block and LAH. A ventricular extrasystole.

XI (A) Flat T waves in I-III and V_{3-6}: Nonspecific changes. Pronounced Q_{III}, as is seen often in obesity. (B) Axis shift to the right in the form of wide and deep S_I. There has developed wide and deep Q_{III}, elevated S-T_{III} and negative T_{III} together with rSr′ pattern in V_1: Incomplete right bundle branch block. The changes in III resemble inferior myocardial infarction, but the over-all pattern is typical of pulmonary embolism; see points (1) and (2), page 75. This is confirmed by the fact that (C) the changes are already regressing on the next day: Smaller S in I and Q in III and the incomplete bundle branch block has disappeared. However, there still are some changes, now also inverted T waves in V_{1-3}; cf. point (3), page 75.
Conclusion: Pulmonary embolism.

XII The first 6 beats show sinus rhythm with slow and decreasing rate. The rate becomes so slow that a junctional center takes over the control of the ventricles from and with beat no. 7, but there must be retrograde block, as the P rhythm continues (in the beginning just before QRS, later hidden within QRS), but cannot conduct antegrade, since the P impulses reach the ventricles in the refractory phase each time. The sinus rhythm again becomes more rapid at the end of strip 1 and takes over activation of the ventricles (the last two beats in strip 1 and the first in strip 2). From here there again is slower sinus rhythm, so that the junctional rhythm can control the ventricles in the remainder of strip 2.
Conclusion: Sinus arrhythmia with idiojunctional rhythm and atrioventricular dissociation ("isorhythmic") during the sinus bradycardia periods.

XIII After five beats with sinus bradycardia with a rate of about 40/min, the entire P-QRS-T complexes in several places arrive at almost twice the basic interval: Second degree sinoatrial block. After beat no. 3 in strip 2 there is third degree sinoatrial block or sinus arrest, which lasts until the two junctional escape beats at the beginning of strip 3 (no preceding P waves). After this, the sinus rhythm starts again with increasing rate.
Conclusion: Second and third degree sinoatrial block.

XIV The ventricular rhythm is irregular. The P rhythm is a regular sinus rhythm with a rate about 105/min. The P-R interval increases through some beats, after which one beat is not conducted at all, i.e., Wenckebach periods (with 4:3 atrioventricular block). QRS is of normal duration, there is left axis deviation, *but because of* the wide, deep Q waves in III and II. There is at the same time a wide, deep Q in V_6. The S-T segment in III is elevated and to a lesser degree also in II and in V_{3-6} with flat T waves in III, II and V_6. The pattern is typical for acute inferolateral infarction and also shows the not altogether rare condition in posterior infarction, that the R waves are relatively tall in the right precordial leads.

Conclusion: Acute inferolateral and posterior myocardial infarction with second degree atrioventricular block (of Mobitz type I).

XV Beat no. 3 is a ventricular extrasystole of "R on T type." It is followed on the S-T segment by a retrograde P wave (positive in this M lead, where the P waves of the sinus rhythm are negative). The compensatory beat (no. 5) shows slight aberrant ventricular conduction.

Conclusion: Ventricular extrasystole with retrograde conduction to the atria and slight post-extrasystolic aberrant conduction.

XVI After beat no. 5, a tachycardia commences with a rate about 185/min with QRS of narrow supraventricular shape, all QRS complexes preceded by P waves of slightly deviant shape with P-R > 0.12 second.

Conclusion: Paroxysmal atrial tachycardia.

XVII Beats nos. 1, 2, 4 and 5 are sinus beats with lengthened P-R = 0.24-0.26 second. Beat no. 3 is a ventricular extrasystole of "R on T type." Beat no. 6 is an end-diastolic ventricular extrasystole from another focus, followed by yet another ventricular extrasystole, which becomes of "R on T type" in relation to beat no. 6, and triggers ventricular fibrillation.

Conclusion: Multifocal ventricular extrasystoles of "R on T type" and in pairs, with ventricular fibrillation after a pair.

XVIII The sequence resembles coupled ventricular premature beats. Closer examination, however, shows that the P rhythm arrives independently of the ventricular beats with a rate of about 125/min. At the beginning of the wide, bizarre ventricular beats, a small, peaked downward-directed impulse is seen: an artificial pacemaker impulse,

171

which is small in this M lead. The pacemaker impulse arrives each time 0.90 second after the patient's own ventricular beats (the narrow QRS complexes).

Conclusion: Third degree atrioventricular block with idiojunctional rhythm and well-functioning (QRS-inhibited) demand pacemaker. The "escape interval" of the pacemaker = 0.90 second.

XIX Bradycardia about 35/min. QRS is not increased in width and is followed immediately by a P wave of "retrograde shape": Junctional rhythm. Left axis deviation (but hardly LAH, as the axis is only about $-30°$; cf. p. 55 and **12,** p. 40). Lengthened Q-T (lead II: Q-T$_c$ = $0.7/\sqrt{1.73}$ = 0.53).

Conclusion: Junctional rhythm. Left axis deviation. Lengthened Q-T interval.

XX The QRS complexes come in groups. In each group an increasing P-R interval is seen, until a single P wave is not conducted: Wenckebach periods.

Conclusion: Second degree atrioventricular block, Mobitz type I.

XXI Sinus rhythm with tachycardia, 110/min in I-III. QRS complexes deformed with QS waves in V$_{4-5}$ and low R waves compared with the Q waves in I, II and V$_6$. S-T segment is elevated, followed by negative T wave of sharp, "coronary" shape in I(,II) and V$_{4-6}$. The S-T elevation in V$_{2-3}$ is within normal limits. Q-T$_c$ (in V$_{4-6}$) = $0.36/\sqrt{0.58}$ = 0.475, lengthened.

Conclusion: Acute anterior infarction (anterolateral), sinus tachycardia, lengthened Q-T interval.

XXII The only striking feature in this electrocardiogram – in addition to the low T waves in the standard leads – is the short Q-T interval; see particularly V$_{2-3}$, where the S wave goes directly over into the T wave.

Conclusion: Short Q-T (the patient had hyperparathyroidism, serum calcium = 19 mg/100 ml).

XXIII There are P waves of normal ("antegrade") shape, but short P-R interval, < 0.12 second. QRS complexes are increased in width, but of a striking shape with a slurred initial component, which, with a bend or notch, goes over into the final part: "delta waves"; cf. page 119.

Conclusion: W-P-W syndrome.

172

XXIV The sinus beats (nos. 1, 2, 3, 6 and 7) show prolonged P-R interval = 0.31 second. Beats nos. 4 and 5 are ventricular extrasystoles from two foci; the first occurs in end-diastole (cf. **98,** p. 97).
Conclusion: Multifocal ventricular extrasystoles. First degree atrioventricular block.

XXV Totally irregular rhythm is seen. The P waves resemble a wavy line in V$_1$: fibrillation waves (f waves) with a mean rate of 570/min at the beginning of V$_1$: atrial fibrillation. QRS shows the shape of an incomplete right bundle branch block: rSR' in V$_1$ and duration 0.11 second. Beats nos. 4 and 5 presumably also are conducted beats, but show aberrant ventricular conduction. They show complete right bundle branch block pattern and terminate short R-R intervals; cf. **92,** page 95.
Conclusion: Atrial fibrillation with varying ventricular response, incomplete right bundle branch block. Presumably two beats with aberrant ventricular conduction.

XXVI Beats nos. 1, 2, 5, 7, 8 and 10 are sinus beats; no. 7 shows aberrant conduction within the ventricles: Normal P and P-R and right bundle branch block. Beats nos. 3, 6 and 9 are premature beats of supraventricular but slightly deviant shape: Supraventricular extrasystoles (atrial or junctional). Beat no. 4 is a ventricular extrasystole (premature and broad, bizarre).
Conclusion: Multiple, multifocal extrasystoles. A beat with aberrant conduction.

XXVII After three sinus beats with decreasing rate, an idioventricular center appears with a rate of 51/min. The last beat in strip 1 and the first two in strip 2 are idioventricular; beat no. 4 in strip 1 is a fusion beat (simultaneous activation of the ventricles from the sinoatrial node and the idioventricular focus). As the P rate again becomes more rapid, sinus rhythm again is obtained (the last three beats). In the period with idioventricular rhythm there is atrioventricular dissociation; see page 23.
Conclusion: Accelerated idioventricular rhythm (cf. **120,** p. 107).

XXVIII After three sinus beats there is a premature beat with a slightly deviant P wave: An atrial extrasystole. After this, the P rhythm continues without QRS complexes: Third degree atrioventricular block with ventricular standstill. After 5½ seconds there is a ventricular beat:

A ventricular escape beat.

Conclusion: Attack of third degree atrioventricular block with ventricular arrest and ventricular escape beat.

XXIX There is in all leads sinus rhythm with normal P-R interval, but in V_{4-6} there is pronounced sinus arrhythmia (the longest P-P interval here is 0.33 second longer than the shortest). Slightly tall $P_{II} = 0.3$ mV. There is right axis deviation and pronounced hypertrophy of the right ventricle (tall R in V_1 and deep S in V_{5-6}), without strain pattern.

Conclusion: Right axis deviation and right ventricular hypertrophy. Sinus arrhythmia. Right atrial enlargement? (child with congenital isolated pulmonary stenosis and respiratory arrhythmia).

XXX There is purely negative deflection (a QS wave) in V_4 and perhaps in V_3 (here there is a doubtful initial R wave in the first complex). The S-T segment is strongly elevated in V_{4-5} and less pronounced in V_3 and V_6 (and suggested in I and II).

Conclusion: Acute anterior infarction (anteroapical).

XXXI Normal electrocardiogram.

XXXII There is arrhythmia. In leads I-III, the 2d and 6th beats are extrasystoles, in V_{1-2}, the 4th and 6th beats and in V_3 the 4th beat. In V_{4-6} there is regularity in the arrhythmia, as every sinus beat is followed by an extrasystole: Coupled extrasystoles (beats nos. 2, 4, 6 and 8) with bigeminy. All extrasystoles are ventricular (wide with a deviant shape without preceding P wave). The QRS complexes of the sinus rhythm show lengthened duration = 0.16 second with configuration of left bundle branch block: Almost exclusively S waves in V_1, only R waves in V_6. The S-T segments and T waves show the "strain-like" pattern usual for left bundle branch block. Q-T interval is lengthened, $Q-T_c = 0.43/\sqrt{0.80} = 0.48$ second.

Conclusion: Left bundle branch block. Many ventricular extrasystoles, periodically (V_{4-6}) coupled with bigeminy. Lengthened duration of systole (Q-T).

XXXIII Beats nos. 3 and 7 are extrasystoles of supraventricular (narrow) shape. They are not preceded by P waves and thus are junctional. There must be retrograde block to the atria, as the P waves of the sinus rhythm continue unchanged (the *antegrade* P waves fall just

after the QRS of the extrasystole).
Conclusion: Junctional extrasystoles of "main stem" type.

XXXIV There is severe sinus bradycardia (beats nos. 1, 3, 5 and 7). The intervals are so long that ventricular escape beats appear in their last part (wide, bizarre ventricular beats nos. 2, 4 and 6).
Conclusion: Sinus bradycardia with ventricular escape beats.

XXXV After two sinus beats, a tachycardia starts with wide, bizarre complexes, the sequence of which does *not* start with any P wave. The rhythm is slightly irregular, rate about 170/min. The attack stops spontaneously: Sinus rhythm in the last three beats.
Conclusion: Paroxysmal ventricular tachycardia.

XXXVI The first five beats are idioventricular (wide, bizarre) with a mean rate of 77/min. The sinus rhythm is very slow and is also seen in the idioventricular rhythm:

P waves are very small but may be seen faintly between the 1st and 2d beats and between the 3d and 4th beats. There thus is atrioventricular dissociation in this segment. After the idioventricular rhythm has stopped, the first P wave is not conducted but the following two are conducted. There thus is severe sinus bradycardia throughout.
Conclusion: Severe sinus bradycardia with a period with accelerated idioventricular rhythm (compare **120,** p. 107).

XXXVII The P rhythm is slow and independent of the patient's own idioventricular beats (QRS nos. 1, 3, 5 and 7). The pacemaker is not inhibited by these and therefore functions as a fixed-rate pacemaker. However, it also fails in this function, as only every second impulse of the pacemaker (the sharp, vertical lines) initiates QRS complexes (beats nos. 2, 4, 6 and 8).
Conclusion: Implanted demand pacemaker with failing functions.

XXXVIII On closer examination, it is seen that there must be a constant P rhythm with a rate of about 115/min. The ventricles are activated from various ventricular centers with irregular rhythm.

Conclusion: Third degree atrioventricular block with irregular idio-ventricular rhythm.

INDEX

177

182